Nutrition: A Very Short Introduction

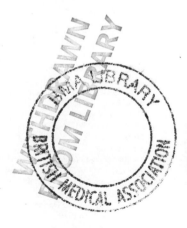
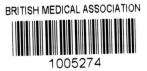

Titles in the series include the following:

David A. Bender

NUTRITION

A Very Short Introduction

OXFORD
UNIVERSITY PRESS

OXFORD
UNIVERSITY PRESS

Great Clarendon Street, Oxford, ox2 6dp,
United Kingdom

Oxford University Press is a department of the University of Oxford.
It furthers the University's objective of excellence in research, scholarship,
and education by publishing worldwide. Oxford is a registered trade mark of
Oxford University Press in the UK and in certain other countries

First edition published in 2014
Impression: 6

Published in the United States of America by Oxford University Press
198 Madison Avenue, New York, NY 10016, United States of America

British Library Cataloguing in Publication Data
Data available

Library of Congress Control Number: 2014931221

ISBN 978-0-19-968192-1

Printed in Great Britain by
Ashford Colour Press Ltd, Gosport, Hampshire

Contents

Acknowledgements

I am grateful to Gary Bateson, Kenneth Bodman, and Carol Farguson, three dear friends who are not nutritionists but have, in their different ways, an interest in food, for their helpful comments on the first draft of this book, as well as to Latha Menon, my editor at Oxford University Press.

List of illustrations

List of tables

Chapter 1
Why eat?

A healthy adult eats about a tonne of food a year. This book attempts to answer the question *why?*—and it does this by exploring the need for food and the uses to which that food is put in the body. Clearly, we eat because we are hungry. However, why have we evolved such complex physiological and psychological mechanisms to control not only hunger and satiety, but also our appetite for different types of food? Why do meals form such an important part of our life?

There is an obvious need for energy from food to perform physical work. Work has to be done to lift a load against the force of gravity and there must be a source of energy to perform that work. As will be discussed in Chapter 2, the energy used in various activities can be measured, as can the energy yield of the foods that provide the fuel for that work. Fats, carbohydrates, protein, and alcohol all provide metabolic fuels.

Apart from its role as a metabolic fuel, there is a requirement for protein in the diet. In a growing child this need is obvious. As the child grows, and the size of its body increases, so there is an increase in the total amount of protein in the body. Adults also require protein in the diet, because there is a continual turnover of body proteins, which have to be replaced. Protein nutrition will be discussed in Chapter 3.

In addition to metabolic fuels and protein, the body has a requirement for two groups of nutrients that are required in very much smaller amounts—the micronutrients, minerals and vitamins. If a metal or ion has a function in the body, it must be provided by the diet, since it is not possible to convert one chemical element into another. The vitamins are organic compounds with a variety of functions. They cannot be synthesized in the body, and so must be provided by the diet. Micronutrients will be discussed in Chapter 7.

Other compounds in the diet (especially from fruit and vegetables) are not dietary essentials, but they may have beneficial effects in reducing the risk of developing a variety of chronic diseases. These compounds will also be discussed in Chapter 7.

The need for water

The body's first need is for water. The human body contains about 60 per cent water—a total of 42 litres in a 70 kg (11 st) person. We excrete water in our urine as a way of ridding the body of the end-products of metabolism, and so we obviously need an intake of water to balance losses from the body. It is possible to survive for several weeks without any food, by using body reserves of fat and protein, but without water, death from dehydration occurs within a few days. There is no storage of water in the body; if water intake is in excess of what is required to maintain the normal levels in the blood stream, cells, and tissues any excess is rapidly lost in the urine. Daily fluid balance for adults is shown in Table 1.

Average daily output of urine is often said to be 1.5 litres (although the figures in Table 1 show that this is an over-estimate), and advertisements for bottled water suggest that we should drink at least this much water per day. At first glance it might seem obvious that we would need an intake of the same amount of fluid to replace the loss in urine. However, as shown in Table 1, total

2

Table 1. Daily fluid balance

		Adult man		Adult woman	
		ml/day	% of total	ml/day	% of total
Intake	fluids	1,950	65	1,400	67
	water in food	700	23	450	21
	metabolic water	350	12	250	12
	total	3,000		2,100	
Output	urine	1,400	47	1,000	48
	sweat	650	22	420	20
	exhaled air	320	11	320	15
	insensible losses through the skin	530	17	270	13
	water in faeces	100	3	90	4
	total	3,000		2,100	

From data reported by W. S. Snyder, M. J. Cook, E. S. Nassett, L. R. Karkhausen, G. Parry-Howells and I. H. Tipton (1975). International Commission on Radiological Protection, *Report of the Task Group on Reference Man*, Pergamon Press, Oxford

Why eat?

daily fluid output from the body is about 3 litres for an adult man and about 2.1 litres for a woman; urine accounts for less than half of this. Equally, fluid consumption in beverages accounts for only about two-thirds of total fluid intake.

In addition to the obvious water in beverages, food provides a significant amount of water: around 22 per cent of total intake, and more if you eat the recommended five servings of fruit and vegetables per day. Most fruits and vegetables contain 60–90 per cent water.

A further source of water is metabolic water—the water produced when fats, carbohydrates, and proteins are oxidized to yield energy. This accounts for about 12 per cent of total water 'intake', and more on a high fat diet, or when metabolizing fat reserves. The camel is able to survive for a considerable time in desert conditions without drinking because it metabolizes the fat stored in its hump; the water produced in fat oxidation meets its needs.

Urine accounts for less than half the total fluid output from the body; as shown in Table 1, the remainder is made up of sweat, water in exhaled air, so-called insensible losses through the skin (this is distinct from the loss in sweat produced by sweat glands), and a relatively small amount in faeces. This last will also increase on a diet rich in fruit and vegetables, because of their content of dietary fibre. Part of the beneficial effect of a high fibre diet is that the fibre retains water in the intestinal tract, so softening the faeces.

Sweat losses obviously depend on the environmental temperature and the intensity of physical activity; we do indeed need to drink more in a hot environment or after strenuous exercise. Losses in exhaled air, faeces, and other insensible losses are relatively constant; urine output varies widely, depending on how much fluid has been consumed. Although average urine volume is 1–1.4 litres per day, this reflects average fluid intake; the output of urine required to ensure adequate excretion of waste material and maintain fluid balance without becoming dehydrated is no more than about 500 ml. Put simply, the more you drink, the more urine you will produce.

A final consideration is whether water is the most appropriate liquid to drink to balance large losses in sweat after vigorous exercise or in a hot climate. The answer is probably no. Sweating involves loss of mineral salts as well as water, and these losses have to be made good. Sports drinks contain balanced mixtures of mineral salts in the same proportions as they are lost in sweat, together, usually, with glucose or another carbohydrate as a source of metabolic fuel and to increase the absorption of mineral salts. Milk and fruit juices also provide mineral salts.

Hunger, satiety, and appetite

Human beings have evolved an elaborate system of physiological mechanisms to ensure that the body's needs for metabolic fuels and nutrients are met, and to balance food intake with energy expenditure. The physiological systems for the control of appetite interact with psychological, social, environmental, and genetic factors, all of which have to be understood in order to understand eating behaviour.

There are hunger centres in the brain (in the hypothalamus) that stimulate us to begin eating, and satiety centres that signal us to stop eating when hunger has been satisfied. Damage to, or destruction of, the hunger centres leads to more or less complete loss of appetite, while electrical stimulation leads to feeding even if the person has eaten enough. Similarly, destruction of the satiety centres leads to uncontrolled eating, and electrical stimulation leads to cessation of feeding, even in someone who is physiologically hungry and in the fasting state.

These appetite control centres have links to other brain regions. The amygdala controls learnt food behaviour—in other words, knowing that something is a food, as opposed to non-food. A young child will put almost anything into its mouth, and gradually learns what is, and what is not, food. Another structure deep in the brain, the nucleus acumbens is part of the reward system of the brain, and is concerned with the pleasure of eating and rewards from food. The appetite control centres also have connections to the cortex and other higher brain centres, which mean that psychological factors (including individual likes and dislikes) can over-ride physiological control of appetite.

The appetite centres respond to the different patterns of metabolic fuels in the bloodstream in the fed and fasting states, and also to hormones such as insulin (which is secreted by the pancreas as blood glucose rises) and glucagon (which is secreted by the pancreas when blood glucose falls), as well as to a number of hormones secreted by the gastro-intestinal tract. One of these hormones, ghrelin, which is secreted by the stomach, acts to increase appetite and stimulate feeding; the others, which are secreted mainly by the small intestine, act as satiety signals, telling us we have eaten enough.

The appetite centres control food intake remarkably precisely. Without conscious effort, most people regulate their food intake to match energy expenditure very closely—they neither waste away from lack of metabolic fuel for physical activity nor lay down excessively large reserves of fat. Even people who have excessive reserves of body fat, and can be considered to be so overweight or obese as to be putting their health at risk, balance their energy intake and expenditure relatively well. The average intake is a tonne of food a year, while the record obese people weigh about 250–300 kg (39–47 st), compared with average weights between 60–100 kg (9–16 st), and it takes many years to achieve such a weight. A gain or loss of 5 kg (11 lb) body weight over 6 months would require only a 1 per cent daily mismatch between food intake and energy expenditure.

In addition to the immediate control of feeding by sensations of hunger and satiety, there is long-term regulation of food intake and energy expenditure. This is a function of the hormone leptin, which is secreted mainly by adipose tissue, where the fat reserves of the body are contained. The circulating concentration of leptin is determined mainly by the amount of adipose tissue (fat) in the body, so that leptin acts as a signal of the size of body fat reserves. In women, low levels of leptin, reflecting adipose tissue reserves that are not adequate to permit a normal pregnancy, both increase food intake and lead to cessation of ovulation and menstruation. This happens when body weight falls to below about 45 kg (7 st).

In addition to its role in appetite control, leptin also acts to increase energy expenditure and body temperature. It does this by increasing metabolic rate (so-called non-shivering thermogenesis), rather than through shivering and physical activity, and so promotes the loss of adipose tissue.

Appetite

In addition to hunger and satiety, which are basic physiological responses, food intake is controlled by appetite, which is related not only to physiological need but also to the pleasure of eating— flavour, texture, and a variety of social and psychological factors. In addition, we become accustomed to eating at a set time, and the clock can provide a cue to eat.

Taste buds on the tongue can distinguish five basic tastes: salt, savoury, sweet, bitter, and sour, as well as a less well understood ability to taste fat. The ability to taste sweetness, savouriness, and fat permits detection of nutrients; the ability to taste sourness and bitterness permits avoidance of toxins in foods.

Salt (more correctly, the mineral sodium) is essential to life, and wild animals will travel great distances to find a salt lick. Like other animals, human beings have evolved a pleasurable response to salty flavours—this ensures that physiological needs are met. However, there is no shortage of salt in developed countries; indeed average intakes of salt are considerably greater than requirements, and pose a hazard to health.

The sensation of savouriness is distinct from that of saltiness, and is sometimes called *umami* (the Japanese word for 'savoury'). It is largely due to the presence of free amino acids in foods, and permits detection of protein-rich foods. The stimulation of the *umami* receptors of the tongue is the basis of flavour enhancers such as monosodium glutamate, an important constituent of traditional oriental condiments that is often used in manufactured foods.

The other instinctively pleasurable taste is sweetness, which permits the detection of carbohydrates, and hence energy sources. While it is only sugars (and artificial sweeteners) that taste sweet, human beings (and some other animals) secrete the enzyme amylase in saliva, which catalyses the breakdown of a small amount of starch, the major dietary carbohydrate, to sweet-tasting sugars, while the food is being chewed.

The tongue is also sensitive to the taste of free fatty acids, and secretes an enzyme (lipase) that catalyses the breakdown of a small amount of fat in the food in the mouth to yield free fatty acids. This permits the detection of fat-rich foods as an energy source.

Sourness and bitterness are instinctively unpleasant sensations; many of the toxins that occur in foods have a bitter or sour flavour. Learnt behaviour will overcome the instinctive aversion, but this is a process of learning or acquiring tastes, not an innate or instinctive response.

In addition to the sensations of taste provided by the taste-buds on the tongue, a great many flavours can be distinguished by the sense of smell. Some flavours and aromas (fruity flavours, fresh coffee, and, at least to a non-vegetarian, the smell of roasting meat) are pleasurable, tempting people to eat and stimulating appetite. Other flavours and aromas are repulsive, warning us not to eat the food. Again this can be seen as a warning of possible danger—the smell of decaying meat or fish tells us that it is not safe to eat.

Like the acquisition of a taste for bitter or sour foods, a taste for foods with what would seem at first to be an unpleasant aroma or flavour can also be acquired. Here things become more complex—a pleasant smell to one person may be a repulsive one to another. Some people enjoy the smell of cooked cabbage and Brussels sprouts, while others can hardly bear to be in the same room. The durian fruit is a highly prized delicacy in Southeast Asia, yet to the uninitiated it has the unappetizing aroma of sewage or faeces.

Disorders of appetite

Extremely rarely, severe obesity may be due to a genetic failure of the secretion of leptin, insensitivity of the leptin receptor, or a defect in a part of the signalling pathway in response to leptin. However, more commonly, it is the interactions between the higher brain centres and the appetite control centres of the hypothalamus that explain why people eat more than they need, and so become overweight or obese. The physiological control of hunger and satiety can be over-ridden by signals from the reward centres of the brain that increase the pleasure of eating. Obesity will be discussed in Chapter 4.

The more serious eating disorders of anorexia nervosa and bulimia are also due to interactions between higher brain centres and the hunger and satiety centres of the hypothalamus, so that a variety of psychological factors can override the normal sensations of hunger.

Anorexia nervosa is characterized by a very severe restriction of food intake, often coupled with excessive exercise, in a desperate attempt not to gain weight. The anorexic patient is commonly very clever about hiding the condition, eating very little apart from salad stuff, playing with food on the plate rather than eating it, sometimes hiding food under the table to pretend it has been eaten. Most sufferers are adolescent girls, although boys can also develop anorexia, and in some cases it develops for the first time in later life. The anorexic patient frequently has a distorted self-image of her or his body, especially as the physical changes of puberty develop, and many welcome the failure of menstruation that occurs as leptin levels fall (due to a body weight below about 45 kg (7 st)). It is estimated that up to 2 per cent of adolescent girls go through a phase of anorexia. In most cases they can be treated successfully by appropriate sensitive psychological help, but a small number continue to have intermittent problems in their eating behaviour throughout life.

Like anorexia nervosa, the underlying cause of bulimia nervosa is psychological. In addition to severe restriction of food intake much of the time, bulimic patients binge eat, consuming a very large amount of food in a very short time, followed by desperate attempts to lose the food they have consumed by inducing vomiting and taking laxatives and diuretics. Again, adolescent girls are most commonly affected, but unlike anorexic patients, their body weight is often within the normal range. Like anorexia, treatment is by psychological help, although in some cases antidepressant medication is successful.

Why do people eat what they do?

People have different responses to any given taste or flavour. This may be explained in terms of childhood memories, pleasurable or otherwise. An aversion to the smell of a food may protect someone who has a specific allergy or intolerance (although sometimes people have a craving for the foods of which they are intolerant).

Most often we simply cannot explain why some people dislike foods that others eat with great relish.

A number of factors influence why people choose either to eat or not to eat particular foods. These include: the availability and cost of foods; the time taken to prepare and consume food; space to prepare and store food; disability and infirmity; personal likes and dislikes; intolerance or allergy; whether you are eating alone or in company; marketing pressure and advertising; religious and ethical taboos; perceived or real health benefits and risks; having to consume a modified diet for the control of a disease; and illness or medication.

In developed countries the easy availability of food means there is little constraint on choice. There is a wide variety of foods available, and when fruits and vegetables are out of season at home they are imported; frozen, canned, or dried foods are widely available. By contrast, in developing countries the availability of food may be a major constraint on what people choose. Even in developed countries, the cost of food is important, and for the more disadvantaged members of the community, poverty may impose severe constraints on their choice of foods.

Religious and ethical considerations are important in determining the choice of foods. Observant Jews and Muslims will only eat meat from animals that have cloven hooves and chew the cud. The terms *kosher* in Jewish law and *hallal* in Islamic law both mean 'clean'; the meat of other animals, that of scavenging animals, birds of prey, and detritus-feeding fish, is regarded as unclean (*traife* or *haram*, respectively). We now know that many of these forbidden animals carry parasites that can infect human beings, so these ancient prohibitions can be seen to be based on food hygiene.

Hindus will not eat beef. The reason for this is that the cow is far too valuable, as a source of milk and dung (as manure and fuel), and as a beast of burden, for it to be killed as a source of meat.

Many people refrain from eating meat as a result of humanitarian concern for the animals involved, or because of real or perceived health benefits. Vegetarians can be divided into various groups, according to the strictness of their diet: some avoid red meat, but will eat poultry and fish; some specifically avoid beef because of the potential risk of contracting variant Creutzfeld-Jacob disease from BSE-infected animals; pescetarians eat fish, but not meat or poultry; ovo-lacto-vegetarians will consume eggs and milk, but not meat or fish; lacto-vegetarians will consume milk, but not eggs; Vegans will eat only plant foods, and no foods of animal origin.

Many people choose to eat organically produced foods in preference to those produced by conventional or intensive farming methods. Organic foods are plants grown without the use of (synthetic) pesticides, fungicides, or inorganic fertilizers and prepared without the use of preservatives. Foodstuffs must be grown on land that has not been treated with chemical fertilizers, herbicides, or pesticides for at least three years. Organic meat is from animals fed on organically grown crops without the use of growth promoters, with only a limited number of medicines to treat disease, and commonly maintained under traditional, non-intensive, conditions. Within the European Union (EU), foods may be labelled as organic if they contain at least 95 per cent organic ingredients and not more than 0.9 per cent genetically modified ingredients.

People who wish to avoid pesticide, fungicide, and other chemical residues in their food, or genetically modified crops, will choose organic produce. Other people choose organic foods because they believe they are nutritionally superior to conventional produce, or because they have a better flavour. There is little evidence that organic produce is nutritionally superior to that produced by conventional farming, although if organic fruits and vegetables are also slower growing, and possibly lower yielding varieties, they may have a higher nutrient content. Many of the older, slower growing and lower yielding fruits and vegetables have a better flavour than more recently introduced varieties that are grown for their rapid yield of a large crop of uniform size and shape. Flavour does not depend on whether or not they are grown organically, but many organic farmers do indeed grow traditional, more flavourful, varieties.

The nutrient content of the same variety of a fruit or vegetable may vary widely, depending not only on the soil (and any fertilizers used), but also on how much sunlight the plant has received and how frequently it has been watered. The apples from one side of a tree may vary in nutrient content from those on the other side of the same tree. The yield, flavour, and nutrient content of the same crop may vary along the length of a field.

While organic produce is indeed free from chemical residues that may be harmful, there is still a potential hazard. Animal manure is used in organic farming to a very much greater extent than in conventional farming, and unless salad vegetables are washed well, there is a potential risk of food poisoning from bacteria in the manure that remains on the produce.

Foods that are commonly eaten in one area may be little eaten elsewhere, even though they are available, simply because people have not been accustomed to eating them. To a very great extent, eating habits of adults are the continued habits learnt in childhood. Haggis and oat cakes travel south from Scotland as specialty items; black pudding is a staple of northern British breakfasts, but is rare in the southeast of England. Until the 1960s yoghurt was almost unknown in Britain, apart from among a few health food 'cranks' and immigrants from eastern Europe. Many British children believe that fish comes as rectangular fish fingers, while children in inland Spain may eat fish and other seafood three or four times a week. The French mock the British habit of eating lamb with mint sauce—and the average American or British reaction to such French delicacies as frogs' legs and snails

13

is one of horror. The British eat their cabbage well boiled; the Germans and Dutch ferment it to produce *sauerkraut*. American cuisine reflects the rich cultural heritage of immigrants to the USA, and while many American foods such as hamburgers and hot dogs are now common throughout the world, others such as succotash and crullers remain, for the present, (regional) American specialties.

This regional and cultural diversity of foods provides one of the pleasures of travel. As people travel more frequently, and become (perhaps grudgingly) more adventurous in their choice of foods, so they create a demand for different foods at home, and there is an increasing variety of foods available in shops and restaurants.

A further factor that has increased the range of foods available has been immigration of people from a variety of different backgrounds, all of whom have, as they have become established, introduced their traditional foods to their new homelands. It is difficult to realize that in the 1960s there was only a handful of tandoori restaurants in the whole of Britain, that pizza was something seen only in southern Italy and a few specialist restaurants, or that Balti cooking and sushi were unknown until the 1990s.

Some people are naturally adventurous, and will try a new food just because they have never eaten it before. Others are more conservative, and will try a new food only when they see someone else eating it safely and with enjoyment. Others are yet more conservative in their food choices; the most conservative eaters 'know' that they do not like a new food *because* they have never eaten it before.

Foods that are scarce or expensive have a certain appeal that is to do with fashion or style; they are (rightly) regarded as luxuries for special occasions rather than everyday meals. Conversely, foods that are widespread and inexpensive have less appeal. In the 19th century, salmon and oysters were so cheap that the articles of apprentices in London specified that they should not be given salmon more than three times a week, while oysters were eaten by the poor. Through much of the 20th century, salmon was scarce and a prized luxury food; however, fish farming has increased the supply of salmon to such an extent that it is again an inexpensive food. Chicken, turkey, guinea fowl, and trout, which were expensive luxury foods in the 1950s, are now widely available as a result of changes in farming practice, and they form the basis of inexpensive meals. By contrast, fish such as cod, herring, and skate, once the basis of cheap meals, are now becoming scarce and expensive as a result of depletion of fish stocks by over-exploitation.

Human beings are social animals, and meals have important social functions. People eating in a group are likely to eat better, or at least have a wider variety of foods and a more lavish and luxurious meal, than people eating alone. The greater the variety of dishes offered, the more people are likely to eat. As we reach satiety with one food, so another, different, flavour is offered to stimulate our appetite. A number of studies have shown that, faced with only one food, people tend to reach satiety sooner than when a variety of foods is on offer. This is the difference between hunger and appetite—even when we are satiated, we can still 'find room' to try something different. This may have been important in evolutionary terms: to ensure a mixed diet providing a variety of nutrients (and especially vitamins and minerals), rather than relying on a single food to simply meet energy needs.

Conversely, and more importantly, many lonely single people (and especially the bereaved elderly) have little incentive to prepare meals, and little stimulus to appetite. While poverty may be a factor, apathy (and frequently, in the case of widowed men, ignorance) severely limits the range of foods eaten, possibly leading to under-nutrition. When these problems are added to by the problems of ill-fitting dentures (which make eating painful), arthritis (which makes handling many foods difficult), and the difficulty of carrying food home from the shops, it is not surprising that we include the elderly among the vulnerable groups of the population who are at risk of under-nutrition.

Food intolerance is a physiological reaction, not just a dislike of a food. The commonest is intolerance of lactose, the sugar in milk. Lactose intolerant people suffer from painful bloating, abdominal cramps, and diarrhoea when they consume more than a small amount of milk. Food allergy is more complex, and involves the formation of antibodies against a protein in a specific food or group of foods. Allergy to the protein gluten in wheat and other cereals is the basis of coeliac disease, and allergy to peanut proteins can lead to serious, and possibly life-threatening, reactions when nuts are eaten. It is now common for labels on manufactured foods to contain 'allergy information', such as whether or not they contain nuts, or may be contaminated with traces of nuts used elsewhere in the factory. Most supermarkets have an aisle of gluten-free foods suitable for people with coeliac disease.

Sometimes people change their diet to avoid certain foods, because of advice from their doctor or a dietitian, as a means of controlling a disease. A more difficult problem is to persuade healthy people to change their diet (e.g., by reducing fat, sugar, and salt intake, as will be discussed in Chapter 5) in order to reduce their risk of developing heart disease and cancer in later life.

Chapter 2
Energy nutrition

Apart from water, the body's first requirement under all conditions is for a source of energy to perform physical and chemical work. The metabolic fuels to provide this energy are derived from the diet—fats, carbohydrates, protein, and alcohol. For a few hours immediately after a meal the constituents of the meal provide these fuels directly. At the same time, reserves of fat (in adipose tissue) and carbohydrate (in liver and muscle) are laid down for use during the period of fasting between meals.

The need for energy to perform physical work and move the body is obvious. Apart from this obvious work output, even at rest the body has a considerable requirement for energy. Only about one-third of the average person's energy expenditure is for voluntary activity; two-thirds is required for maintenance of the body's functions, metabolic integrity, and homeostasis (maintenance of the normal state) of the internal environment.

This energy requirement at rest is the basal metabolic rate (BMR). Part of this requirement is obvious—the heart beats to circulate the blood, breathing continues, and there is considerable electrical activity in nerves and muscles, whether they are 'working' or not. The brain and nervous system comprise only about 2 per cent of body weight, but consume some 20 per cent of resting energy expenditure, because of the need to maintain electrical activity.

Less obviously, there is also a requirement for energy for the wide variety of biochemical reactions occurring all the time in the body: laying down reserves of fat and carbohydrate; the turnover of tissue proteins; transport of compounds into and out of cells; and the synthesis and secretion of hormones.

Energy expenditure can be measured by the output of heat from the body. The unit of heat used in the early studies was the calorie—the amount of heat required to raise the temperature of 1 gram of water by 1 degree Celsius. The calorie is still used in nutrition, usually as the kilocalorie, kcal (sometimes written as Calorie with a capital C). One kcal is 1,000 calories (10^3 cal), and hence the amount of heat required to raise the temperature of 1 kg of water by 1 degree Celsius.

More correctly, the Joule is used as the unit of energy. The Joule is an SI unit (International System of Units), named after James Prescott Joule (1818–89), who first showed the equivalence of heat, mechanical work, and other forms of energy. In nutrition, the kiloJoule (kJ = 10^3 J) and megaJoule (MJ = 10^6 J) are used.

To convert between calories and Joules:

1 kcal = 4.184 kJ (normally rounded off to 4.2 kJ)
1 kJ = 0.239 kcal (normally rounded off to 0.24 kcal)

The average total daily energy expenditure of adults is between 1,900 to 2,400 kcal (7.5 to 10 MJ) for women and 2,000 to 2,900 kcal (8 to 12 MJ) for men.

Measurement of energy expenditure

Energy expenditure can be measured by measuring heat output from the body, but this is a tedious experimental procedure, requiring a thermally insulated room in which a small increase in temperature can be measured accurately. An indirect method of determining energy expenditure is by measurement of the consumption of oxygen.

It is relatively simple to measure oxygen consumption by sampling inspired and exhaled air and measuring the oxygen content of each—the difference is the amount of oxygen that has been consumed. Using a respirometer (a small back pack containing an air bag attached to a mouthpiece) it is possible to measure oxygen consumption in a variety of different activities, as well as at rest, for periods of an hour or so at a time. Early studies calibrated such measurements of oxygen consumption against direct measurement of heat production and showed that each litre of oxygen consumed is equivalent to energy expenditure of 4.8 kcal (20 kJ).

BMR is determined by measuring oxygen consumption over a period of about hour, with the subject completely at rest (but not asleep), in a comfortably warm room (so that energy is not being expended to maintain body temperature), some four hours after a meal, so that energy is not being expended on digestion, absorption of the products of digestion, or the synthesis of reserves of fat and carbohydrate. If the experimental conditions are not rigorously controlled, it is usual to call the resultant energy expenditure the resting metabolic rate (RMR), keeping the term BMR for studies conducted under precisely controlled conditions. Both BMR and RMR are expressed as kcal (or MJ)/24 hours.

It is important that the person is not asleep when measuring BMR or RMR. Some people show an increase in metabolic rate and become hot when they are asleep, while others show a small drop in body temperature, associated with a reduction in metabolic rate. People whose body temperature falls slightly in sleep are biologically efficient; they are conserving energy. However, those biologically inefficient people whose metabolic rate rises when they are asleep are fortunate in that this increase in metabolic rate means that they are consuming more metabolic fuel. They are increasing their energy expenditure to 'burn off' surplus metabolic fuels they have consumed in food. They do not gain weight as readily as people whose metabolic rate falls when they are asleep.

The energy cost of various types of physical activity can also be determined by measuring oxygen consumption. Although the results of any such measurement will be expressed in kcal (or kJ), it is more useful to express the results as a multiple of the individual's BMR. This means that it is relatively easy to apply the results of studies in a small number of people to others whose BMR can be measured (or estimated from body weight, age, and gender), but whose energy expenditure in physical activity has not been measured. This multiple of BMR for any given physical activity is known as the physical activity ratio (PAR) for that activity, or sometimes as the metabolic equivalent of the task (MET). As shown in Table 2, gentle, sedentary activities have a PAR of up to 1.4 x BMR, while strenuous activities such as walking cross-country with a load may have a PAR of almost 8 x BMR.

If we sum the PARs for the different activities through the day, multiplied by the fraction of the 24 hours spent in each activity, we can calculate a person's overall physical activity level (PAL). Table 3 shows the ranges of PAL for people in light, moderate, and heavy occupational work, calculated through the eight-hour working day, and not allowing for any additional energy expenditure in leisure activities. At first sight, these values of PAL do not seem to fit well with the energy cost (PAR) of individual activities, but most people do not engage in the more strenuous activities for very long, and much of their day is spent in less strenuous activities or at rest.

Measurement (or calculation) of BMR and calculation of a person's PAL does not give his or her total energy expenditure, because we have to add in the metabolic energy cost of eating—the cost of synthesizing and secreting digestive enzymes, absorbing the products of digestion, and, perhaps most importantly, the

Table 2. Physical activity ratios (PARs) (multiples of basal metabolic rate (BMR)) in different types of activity

PAR	
1.0–1.4	*Lying, standing or sitting at rest*: watching tv, reading, writing, eating, playing cards and board games
1.5–1.8	*Sitting:* sewing, knitting, playing piano, driving
	Standing: preparing vegetables, washing dishes, ironing, general office and laboratory work
1.9–2.4	*Standing:* mixed household chores, cooking, playing snooker or bowls
2.5–3.3	*Standing:* dressing, undressing, showering, making beds, vacuum cleaning
	Walking: 3–4 km/h, playing cricket
	Occupational: tailoring, shoemaking, electrical and machine tool industry, painting and decorating
3.4–4.4	*Standing:* mopping floors, gardening, cleaning windows, table tennis, sailing
	Walking: 4–6 km/h, playing golf
	Occupational: motor vehicle repairs, carpentry and joinery, chemical industry, bricklaying
4.5–5.9	*Standing:* polishing furniture, chopping wood, heavy gardening, volley ball
	Walking: 6–7 km/h
	Exercise: dancing, moderate swimming, gentle cycling, slow jogging
	Occupational: labouring, hoeing, road construction, digging and shovelling, felling trees
6.0–7.9	*Walking:* uphill with load or cross-country, climbing stairs
	Exercise: jogging, cycling, energetic swimming, skiing, tennis, football

From data reported by Department of Health (1991). *Dietary Reference Values for Food Energy and Nutrients for the United Kingdom.* HMSO, London; and FAO/WHO/UNU (1985). 'Energy and Protein Requirements: Report of a Joint FAO/WHO/UNU Expert Consultation, WHO Technical Reports Series 724, WHO, Geneva

Energy nutrition

Table 3. Classification of types of occupational work by physical activity ratio (PAR) (multiples of basal metabolic rate (BMR)): figures show the average PAR through an eight-hour working day, excluding leisure activities

Work intensity	PAR[1]	
Light	1.7	professional, clerical, and technical workers, administrative and managerial staff, sales representatives, housewives/-husbands
Moderate	2.2–2.7	sales staff, domestic service, students, transport workers, joiners, roofing workers
Moderately heavy	2.3–3.0	machine operators, labourers, agricultural workers, bricklaying, masonry
Heavy	2.8–3.8	labourers, agricultural workers, bricklayers, masonry workers where there is little or no mechanization

(1) Where a range of PAR is shown, the lower figure is for women and the higher for men

From data reported by Department of Health (1991). *Dietary Reference Values for Food Energy and Nutrients for the United Kingdom*. HMSO, London

energy cost of synthesizing reserves of fat and carbohydrate, and the energy cost of the increase in protein synthesis that occurs after a meal. This is seen as an increase in heat output from the body after eating—diet-induced thermogenesis. Overall it may account for as much as 10 per cent of the energy yield of the meal.

Metabolic fuels

The dietary sources of metabolic energy (the metabolic fuels) are carbohydrates, fats, protein, and alcohol. As can be seen from Table 4, fat yields more than twice as much energy per gram as carbohydrates and proteins.

Table 4. Energy yield and oxygen consumption in oxidation of metabolic fuels

Fuel	Energy yield		Oxygen consumed	Energy yield/ oxygen consumption	
	kJ/g	kcal/g	l/g	kJ/l oxygen	kcal/l oxygen
Carbohydrate	16	4	0.829	~ 20	~5
Protein	17	4	0.966	~ 20	~5
Fat	37	9	2.016	~ 20	~5
Alcohol	29	7	1.691	~ 20	~5

Although there is a requirement for energy sources in the diet, it does not matter unduly how that requirement is met. There is no requirement for a dietary source of carbohydrate because the body can synthesize as much carbohydrate as is needed from the amino acids derived from proteins. Similarly, there is no requirement for a dietary source of fat, apart from the essential fatty acids that are required in relatively small amounts, and there is certainly no requirement for a dietary source of alcohol. Diets that provide more than about 35–40 per cent of energy from fat are associated with increased risk of heart disease and some cancers, and there is some evidence that diets that provide more than about 20 per cent of energy from protein are also associated with chronic diseases. Therefore, the general consensus is that diets should provide about 55 per cent of energy from carbohydrates, 30 per cent from fat, and 15 per cent from protein.

Although there is no requirement for fat in the diet, fats are nutritionally important, for a number of reasons. First, it is difficult to eat enough of a very low-fat diet to meet energy requirements. The problem in many less developed countries, where under-nutrition is common, is that diets provide only 10 to 15 per cent of energy from fat, and it is difficult to consume a sufficient bulk of food to meet energy requirements. By contrast, the problem in Western countries is an undesirably high intake of fat, contributing to the development of obesity and chronic diseases. In addition, four of the vitamins—A, D, E, and K—are fat-soluble, and are found in fatty and oily foods. They are absorbed dissolved in fat, so with a very low-fat diet the intake and absorption of these vitamins may be inadequate to meet requirements. There is a requirement for small amounts of two essential fatty acids that cannot be synthesized in the body and must be provided in the diet. Finally, in many foods a great deal of the flavour (and hence the pleasure of eating) is carried in the fat; also, fat lubricates food, making it easier to chew and swallow.

Metabolic fuels in the fed and fasting states

In the fed state, during three to four hours after eating a meal, the main fuel for muscle and other tissues is glucose, which is produced by the digestion of dietary carbohydrates. Glucose in excess of immediate requirements will be used for synthesis of the storage carbohydrate glycogen in liver and muscle, and also for synthesis of fatty acids, and then fat, in liver and adipose tissue. Dietary fat will mainly be used to add to fat reserves in adipose tissue. Amino acids from dietary protein in excess of requirements for tissue protein synthesis will be used as metabolic fuels, or used to synthesize glucose (and hence glycogen) or fatty acids (and hence fat).

The fasting state begins some four to five hours after a meal, when the body needs to call on the reserves laid down after a meal. Glycogen reserves can provide glucose, but the total amount of glycogen in the body would only last for 12 to 18 hours, and the brain is more or less completely reliant on a source of glucose (while red blood cells are completely reliant on glucose). Muscle can use glucose (from the bloodstream or its own glycogen reserves), but it can also use fatty acids liberated from adipose tissue fat reserves. In the fasting state, muscle ceases to take up glucose from the bloodstream and uses fatty acids as its main fuel, so sparing glucose for the brain and red blood cells. During fasting, the rate of protein synthesis slows down, but breakdown continues at a more or less constant rate. This leads to the liberation of amino acids that can be used in the liver for the synthesis of glucose that can be exported for use by the brain and red blood cells. This is the process of gluconeogenesis, the new synthesis of glucose from non-carbohydrate precursors.

As fasting continues for more than about 12 hours, and muscle reserves of glycogen are more or less exhausted, fatty acids alone cannot meet the needs for muscle metabolism. At this stage, the liver takes up some of the fatty acids that have been liberated from adipose tissue, and uses them to synthesize small water-soluble compounds (the ketone bodies) that can be used by muscle and, to a limited extent, also the brain. Gluconeogenesis from amino acids liberated by protein breakdown continues.

Energy balance

In order to maintain a constant body weight, it is necessary to balance energy intake from food with energy expenditure. Most people achieve this balance very well, and indeed, as noted earlier, even grossly overweight people are in energy balance, with a stable, if excessive, body weight. Part of this ability to balance energy intake and expenditure is the result of the physiological systems of control over hunger, satiety, and appetite discussed in Chapter 1. In addition, there are physiological mechanisms that permit the metabolism of metabolic fuels not linked to the normal conservation of energy in the form of ATP (adenosine triphosphate). ATP is the 'energy currency' of the cell, and is used: to power chemical reactions; to transport compounds into and out of cells; in electrical activity of brain and nerves; and in contraction of muscle for movement and physical work. The processes of oxidation of metabolic fuels linked to the formation of ATP are normally tightly coupled, so that metabolic fuels are only oxidized when there is a need for ATP. However, there are proteins in muscle and some other tissues that can uncouple these reactions to some extent. This uncoupling is important in response to exposure to cold, as a means of generating heat to maintain body temperature. It is usually referred to as non-shivering thermogenesis, as opposed to shivering when increased muscle contraction leads to increased heat production. The increase in body temperature and metabolic rate that some people show when they are asleep is the result of such uncoupling of fuel oxidation and ATP formation.

If you deliberately overfeed someone by 10 per cent, they will gain weight initially, then stabilize at a higher body weight. Initially they will be in positive energy balance, with an intake greater than their expenditure, and laying down additional reserves of body fat. When their weight has stabilized, they will return to balance, despite still eating 10 per cent more than previously, at a higher body weight. There are four reasons for this. If you eat more food, there is a greater energy cost for digestion and absorption, and the synthesis of fat and carbohydrate reserves—an increase in diet-induced thermogenesis. As the amount of adipose tissue in the body increases, there is an increase in the secretion of the hormone leptin, which acts to increase the uncoupling of fuel oxidation and ATP formation, resulting in increased oxidation of metabolic fuels. As body weight increases, so there is an increase in BMR, and more importantly, as body weight increases, so the energy cost of moving that body increases, so that the energy cost of physical activity increases.

Conversely, if you underfeed someone by 10 per cent, they will initially lose weight, then come back into energy balance at a lower body weight. The reasons for this are the converse of those for the re-establishment of energy balance at a higher body weight with overfeeding. If less food is eaten, there will be a lower energy cost of digesting and absorbing that food, and a lower energy cost of synthesizing fat and carbohydrate reserves. As the amount of adipose tissue in the body falls, so there is a reduction in the secretion of leptin, a reduction in non-shivering thermogenesis, and a reduction in the oxidation of metabolic fuels not linked to the formation and utilization of ATP. Finally, as body weight falls, there is a reduction in BMR, and the energy cost of moving a smaller, lighter, body is less, so the energy cost of physical activity decreases.

Physical activity and exercise

A desirable level of physical activity for cardiovascular and respiratory fitness is about $1.7 \times$ BMR. This should be easy to achieve with normal physical activity, but fewer than a quarter of adults in most developed countries do so, and, as discussed in Chapter 4, a major contributor to the worldwide epidemic of obesity is a sedentary lifestyle, with relatively low physical activity.

It is obvious from the figures in Table 2 that energy expenditure increases with the intensity of physical activity. What is less obvious is that the pattern of metabolic fuels used also changes. In moderate exercise, muscle is well oxygenated and uses mainly fatty acids (either from free fatty acids and lipids in the bloodstream or from its own reserves of fat laid down between muscle fibres) as its main fuel. As the intensity of exercise increases, so the need for metabolism of metabolic fuels by muscle exceeds the rate at which oxygen can enter the muscle cells. This is the so-called aerobic threshold—muscle will continue to metabolize as much fat as the available oxygen permits, and will meet the increased demand by anaerobic metabolism of glucose. This is a relatively inefficient process that leads to the release of lactic acid from muscle. This lactic acid will later be taken up by the liver and used for resynthesis of glucose. The synthesis of glucose from lactic acid requires ATP, and as a result there is an increase in metabolic rate and oxygen consumption after exercise (so-called oxygen debt) as some of the lactic acid is oxidized completely to provide the ATP needed for glucose synthesis.

This change in fuel utilization by muscle with increasing intensity of exercise means that if the main aim of exercising is to lose excess fat, a relatively prolonged period of low intensity exercise is better than a short period of intense exercise. One cynic has suggested that walking a mile each way to and from the gym, and not going in, is better than driving to the gym and exercising intensely for a short time. Certainly it is easy to increase physical activity without engaging in formal exercise, for example by walking or cycling rather than driving, or using stairs instead of lifts and escalators.

Chapter 3
Protein nutrition

About 14 per cent of the human body is protein, so it is obvious that a growing child must have an intake of protein to allow for an increase in the total amount of protein in the body as it grows. Similarly, a pregnant woman obviously needs an intake of protein to permit the fetus to grow. What is less obvious is why an adult, whose body weight does not change, nevertheless requires protein in the diet.

Nitrogen balance and protein requirements

Studies in the 19th century showed that animals that were fed a protein-free diet could not maintain their body weight, but wasted away. Proteins contain the element nitrogen in their constituent amino acids, and a chemical method for measuring total nitrogen-containing compounds in the diet, and in urine and faeces was developed by Johan Kjeldahl in 1883—a method that is still in use today. This made it possible to investigate the balance between protein intake and excretion of the products of protein metabolism, and so to begin to estimate how much protein is required in the diet.

Nitrogen balance is the difference between the intake of nitrogen-containing compounds in the diet (mainly protein), and the excretion of nitrogen-containing compounds (mainly small molecules such as urea) from the body. An adult is normally in nitrogen balance or nitrogen equilibrium—the intake and excretion of nitrogenous compounds are equal and there is no change in the total amount of protein in the body. A growing child, a pregnant woman, or someone who is recovering from protein loss is in positive nitrogen balance—the excretion of nitrogen-containing compounds is less than the intake. In this case, there is retention of nitrogen-containing compounds (as protein) in the body, and an increase in the total protein content of the body.

Studies of nitrogen balance are still used to determine protein requirements. If someone is fed too little protein, they will not be able to maintain nitrogen equilibrium. Their excretion of nitrogen-containing compounds will be greater than their intake, and there will be a loss of body protein. This is negative nitrogen balance, and is also seen in response to trauma or infection, and in patients with advanced cancer.

Protein requirements are determined by feeding volunteers on different levels of protein intake, and measuring their nitrogen balance. If they are fed 20–30g of protein per day at the start of the experiment, they will be unable to maintain nitrogen balance. Their protein intake is then increased gradually (with time to adapt to each change in intake) until they can maintain equilibrium between intake and excretion. This intake is just meeting their requirement. As their intake is increased above their requirement level, initially they have a period of positive nitrogen balance while they replace the protein that was lost when their intake was inadequate. Once the lost protein has been replaced, they remain in nitrogen equilibrium. Eating a high protein diet does not increase the total amount of protein in the body, but breakdown or catabolism of protein increases, and the excretion of nitrogen-containing compounds increases, to match the intake.

The outcome of studies on nitrogen balance is that the average protein requirement for an adult is 0.65g of protein/kg body weight, or 45.5g of protein per day for a 70kg (11 st) person. There is individual variation around this average requirement, and in order to ensure that essentially everyone's protein requirements are met, an appropriate level of protein intake is set at 2 x standard deviation above the average requirement. This gives a safe and adequate level of protein intake as 0.83 g/kg body weight, or 58g (2 oz) of protein/day for a 70kg (11 st) person. Average intakes of protein in developed countries are considerably higher than this—of the order of 90g (3½ oz)/day, so there is unlikely to be a problem of protein deficiency.

An alternative way of expressing protein requirements is to calculate the percentage of energy intake coming from protein, which yields 4 kcal (17 kJ)/gram. On this basis, the safe and adequate level of protein intake represents about 8.25 per cent of energy intake, and average Western diets provide 14–15 per cent of energy from protein. Even in developing countries, it is likely that protein intake as a percentage of energy intake will be adequate to meet an adult's needs. Apart from cassava, yam, and rice, most starchy dietary staple foods provide more than 9 per cent of energy from protein, and it would only need a relatively small amount of meat, fish, or another protein-rich food to ensure an adequate intake.

Dynamic equilibrium and the need for dietary protein

It was not until the middle of the 20th century that the underlying reason for the need for an intake of protein in an adult became apparent. Rudolph Schönheimer fed animals diets containing amino acids labelled with a stable isotope as part of their protein intake. Since the animals were in nitrogen equilibrium, he expected to recover almost all of the isotopic label in urine and faeces. In fact he recovered less than half—the remainder was incorporated into tissue proteins. Although the total amount of protein in the body remained unchanged, there is continual breakdown of tissue proteins and replacement by newly synthesized protein. Schönheimer coined the term 'dynamic equilibrium' for this process.

We now know that different proteins in the body are broken down and replaced at different rates. Some, and especially enzymes that are control points in metabolic pathways, are broken down and replaced within a few hours; others, which can be considered to be 'housekeeping' enzymes and structural proteins turn over more slowly, with a half-life of days or weeks. Collagen, the structural protein of bones and connective tissue has a half-life of almost a year.

Studies with stable isotopically labelled amino acids have also shown that although an adult is overall in nitrogen equilibrium, this represents the average of periods of negative balance between meals and positive balance after a meal.

In the fasting state (starting about 4 to 5 hours after a meal), the rate of protein synthesis slows down. This is because protein synthesis is very energy expensive, and in the fasting state we are reliant on reserves of fat and carbohydrate laid down after a meal as the source of metabolic fuel—for this reason, we need to conserve energy. Protein breakdown continues at the normal rate, liberating amino acids that are not used for replacement protein synthesis, but are metabolized as metabolic fuel or used for glucose synthesis.

After a meal there is an abundant source of metabolic fuel (sufficiently in excess of immediate requirements to permit reserves of fat and carbohydrate to be laid down in preparation for the interval between meals). There is also an abundant supply of amino acids from protein in the diet. This permits a period of positive nitrogen balance to replace the protein that was broken down in the fasting state. It is this replacement of protein broken down in the fasting state that explains why an adult has a requirement for an intake of protein although overall there is no change in the total body protein content.

Is there a need for protein supplements?

Sportspeople and athletes in training, and especially body builders, are increasing their muscle levels and, therefore, the total amount of protein in their body. Many people think that this means they need more protein in their diet, and this is correct to a certain extent. However, even children recovering from severe malnutrition, who show rapid catch-up growth, the gain in body protein is less than half the total amount of protein that is synthesized and broken down each day. Average intakes of protein are sufficiently in excess of requirements that there is no need for more protein in the diet (whether from eating large amounts of meat or from taking protein supplements) to permit an increase in the total amount of protein in the body as muscle is gained through training. On the other hand, there is a need for increased energy intake to meet both the cost of new protein synthesis and the energy cost of training and increased physical activity. If a person eats a larger quantity of their usual types of food, he or she will automatically increase not only energy but also protein intake.

The protein supplements that are marketed for sportspeople therefore seem to be unnecessary. The American Dietetic Association has stated that an intake of 1.2–1.7g of protein/kg body weight by endurance and strength-trained athletes 'can generally be achieved through diet without the use of protein or amino acid supplements. Energy intake to maintain body weight is necessary for optimal protein use.' There is also concern that some of these supplements may contain undeclared ingredients, including steroid hormones, which may increase tissue protein synthesis, but are banned substances in competitive sport.

The same argument applies to people recovering from a period of illness. They may have lost a considerable amount of body protein, as a result of both surgical trauma and prolonged bed-rest. However, assuming that they can eat enough of their normal foods to meet their energy requirements, they will have sufficient protein to permit replacement protein synthesis during convalescence. Nevertheless, in some cases it may be difficult for a sick person to eat enough food to meet requirements, and a dietitian may well prescribe a high-energy or high-protein supplement.

Not all proteins have the same nutritional value

Proteins are made from 21 different amino acids. Twelve of these can be synthesized in the body from more or less common metabolic intermediates, as long as there is an adequate total amount of protein in the diet. However, the remaining nine cannot be synthesized in the body, but must be provided in the diet. These are called the essential or indispensable amino acids. If they are not provided in adequate amounts to meet the need for tissue protein synthesis then it is not possible to maintain nitrogen equilibrium. Once the essential amino acid that is present in least amount compared with the requirement has been used, the remaining amino acids, both essential and non-essential, will be metabolized as metabolic fuel. Requirements for the essential amino acids can be determined by studies of nitrogen balance, where people are fed adequate amounts of total protein, but with one or other of the essential amino acids in limited amounts, until the intake at which nitrogen equilibrium can just be maintained is found.

Knowing the requirement for each essential amino acid as a percentage of total protein intake allows us to define protein quality. A protein that provides only 50 per cent of the requirement for one of the essential amino acids will have a protein score of only 0.5. A protein that provides more than the requirement of all of the essential amino acids will have a protein score of 1.0. In some countries, food labelling legislation requires that not only must the protein content of a food be declared, but also the quality of that protein, which is expressed as the 'protein score' (also called the 'amino acid score'), corrected for the digestibility of the protein. This is known as the 'protein digestibility corrected amino acid score' (PDCAAS).

Milk and eggs have a protein score of 1 and meat has a score of 0.8–0.9. However, individual plant proteins have a score as low as 0.4–0.5. This has led to a distinction between animal proteins—sometimes called 'first class' proteins—and vegetable proteins—sometimes called 'second class' proteins. While this is so when individual proteins are considered, it makes little or no difference when whole diets are considered. The usability of cereal proteins is limited by their content of the amino acid lysine, but they have a relative excess of the amino acid methionine. By contrast, the usability of the proteins of peas and beans is limited by their content of methionine, and they have a relative excess of lysine. In a judicious mixture of vegetable proteins (e.g. rice and peas, or pasta and beans), the excess amino acids in one protein will compensate for the deficit in the other, and the overall protein score will be 0.8–0.9, the same as that of meat. The protein score of diets in developing countries, with little meat, eggs, fish, or dairy produce, is almost as high as that of diets in Western countries. There is certainly no problem in obtaining sufficient protein, or in overall adequate quality, from a vegetarian diet. Even among omnivores in Western countries, just over one-third of protein intake comes from cereals, fruit, and vegetables.

Chapter 4

Over-nutrition: problems of overweight and obesity

Historically, a high body weight was considered to be desirable. Only wealthy people could afford to eat excessive food and gain body weight, so what we would now call overweight or obesity was a visible sign of wealth and prosperity. In evolutionary terms there was a survival advantage in having sufficient reserves of fat to survive periods of food shortage and famine. However, from the beginning of the 20th century, insurance companies started to collect data on body weight and life expectancy, showing that excessive weight was associated with earlier death, and therefore a poorer risk for life insurance.

Western society's attitude to obesity has changed, and obesity is now considered to be undesirable, and places a considerable financial strain on health services. Fashion emphasizes slimness, often using models who are not just slim, but frankly underweight. Because of this, many overweight and obese people have problems of a poor self-image, and low self-esteem. They are certainly not helped by the all-too-common prejudice against them, the difficulty of buying clothes that will fit, and the fact that they are often regarded as a legitimate butt of crude and cruel jokes. Overweight children are reviled by their leaner peers and are often the subject of bullying. This may lead to a sense of isolation and withdrawal from society, and often will result in increased food consumption, for comfort—resulting in yet more weight gain, a further loss of self-esteem, further withdrawal, and more eating for compensation.

The psychological and social problems of the obese spill over to people of normal weight as well. There is continual advertising pressure for 'slimness', and newspapers and magazines are full of propaganda for slimness, and 'diets' for weight reduction. This may be one of the factors in the development of major eating disorders such as anorexia nervosa and bulimia.

Desirable body weight and body mass index

Data from life insurance companies, then later from prospective studies in which large numbers of people were followed for many years, after being classified by body weight at the beginning of the study, have allowed us to define ranges of desirable and undesirable weight. A person's weight obviously depends on their height. Early tables showed weight for height. However, it is now more usual to use ranges of body mass index (BMI)—the ratio of body weight/height^2 (kg/m^2). This is sometimes called Quetelet's index, after the Belgian mathematician Adolphe Quetelet (1796 –1874) who first calculated it, and showed that it gave an index of weight that was independent of height.

A desirable range of BMI is 20 to 25 kg/m^2. This is associated with optimum life expectancy.

BMI 25 to 30 (about 5 to 15 kg, 10 to 33 lb, over desirable weight for height) is classified as overweight, and is associated with a 10 to 35 per cent increased risk of early death. In some countries the range of BMI 25 to 27 is classified as 'acceptable but not desirable', but still carries a 10 to 15 per cent increased risk of early death.

BMI 30 to 40 (about 15 to 25 kg, 33 to 55 lb, over desirable weight for height) is classified as obesity, and carries a 35 to 135 per cent increased risk of early death. BMI greater than 40 (more than

25 kg, 55 lb, over desirable weight for height) is classified as severe obesity, and carries an even higher risk of early death.

The health risks of obesity

The major causes of early death associated with obesity are cancer (especially breast, prostate, and colorectal cancers); atherosclerosis, coronary heart disease, high blood pressure and stroke; type II diabetes mellitus and its complications; and respiratory diseases. The risk of developing type II diabetes is 20 to 80 times higher in obese people than lean people.

In addition to the diseases caused by, or associated with, obesity, obese people are considerably more at risk of death during surgery and of developing post-operative complications. Surgery takes longer and is more difficult when the surgeon has to cut through large amounts of subcutaneous and intra-abdominal adipose tissue. More importantly, anaesthesia depresses lung function (as does being in a supine position), in all people. Obese people suffer from impaired lung function under normal conditions; because of the burden of fat in the upper part of the body, their total lung capacity may be only 60 per cent of that in lean people, and the workload on the respiratory muscles may be twice that of lean people. Therefore, they are especially at risk during surgery. Because of this impaired lung function, obese people are more at risk of respiratory distress, pneumonia, and bronchitis than are lean people.

Excess body weight is associated with increased morbidity from such conditions as arthritis of the hips and knees, associated with the increased stress on weight-bearing joints, and varicose veins and haemorrhoids. Obesity in childhood and adolescence is associated with lower bone mineral density and increased risk of developing osteoporosis in later life.

These health risks of obesity have serious implications for health services. In the UK it is estimated that treating obesity and its

related diseases costs the National Health Service some £4.2
billion a year—almost 4 per cent of total health service spending.

The distribution of fat is important

There are two types of adipose tissue in the body: subcutaneous
fat reserves under the skin, which is mainly, but not entirely, on
the hips and thighs, and fat within the abdominal cavity, between
the organs, which is mainly seen as increased waist diameter or
waist:hip ratio.

Subcutaneous fat acts mainly as a reserve of metabolic fuel and is
relatively metabolically inactive. By contrast, intra-abdominal
adipose tissue is metabolically more active, and releases fatty acids
directly to the liver, where they stimulate the production of
glucose, whether or not there is a need for increased blood
glucose. Intra-abdominal adipose tissue also secretes hormones
that antagonize the actions of insulin, so leading to the
development of type II diabetes.

In evolutionary terms, intra-abdominal adipose tissue developed
to metabolize fatty acids as a means of maintaining body
temperature, and was originally the very metabolically active
brown adipose tissue—so called because it has a red-brown
colour, while storage adipose tissue is white or pale yellow.
However, in response to a high fat diet (and the reduced need
for heat production when we have better heating in homes) it
has differentiated into storage adipose tissue, but continues
to be more metabolically active than subcutaneous
adipose tissue.

While there is no doubt that any excess body fat is a cause of ill
health and premature death, intra-abdominal adipose tissue is
considerably more hazardous than subcutaneous fat.
Measurement of waist circumference gives an indication of
intra-abdominal adipose tissue; desirable sizes are waist

circumference less than 102 cm (40 inches) for men or less than 88 cm (35 inches) for women.

The obesity epidemic

Over the past half century there has been a considerable increase in the prevalence of obesity in all developed countries. In 1980, 39 per cent of men and 32 per cent of women in Britain had a BMI above 25, and 6 per cent of men and 8 per cent of women were clinically obese with a BMI above 30. This was sufficiently worrying for the Department of Health to set a goal in its 'The Health of the Nation' policy document to halve obesity within a decade. In fact, by 1991, 53 per cent of men and 64 per cent of women had a BMI above 25, and 13 per cent of men and 16 per cent of women were clinically obese. By 2003, 67 per cent of men and 60 per cent of women had a BMI over 25, and 24 per cent of men and 26 per cent of women were clinically obese. There was a three-fold increase in obesity in 23 years. The encouraging news is that since 2003 there seems to have been little further increase, although it is not clear whether this is the result of health promotion activities by general practitioners and the Department of Health, or whether it reflects the premature death of overweight and obese people.

There has also been an increase in the numbers of overweight and obese children. In 1995, 24 per cent of boys and 25 per cent of girls ages between 2 to 15 were overweight or obese; 10.9 per cent of boys and 12 per cent of girls were obese. By 2006, this had increased to 30.6 per cent of boys and 28.7 per cent of girls being overweight or obese, and 17.3 per cent of boys and 14.7 per cent of girls being obese. There is some good news here, in that the levels of overweight and obesity among children peaked in 2004, and showed a small decrease from this peak by 2006 (the most recent date for which figures are available). Since premature death is not the problem for overweight children, this suggests that the health promotion activities to target children are having some success.

Britain is not alone in this. All developed countries have seen similar increases in overweight and obesity, although the increases started earlier in the USA and some other countries than in the UK, and later in other countries. In most developing countries, where undernutrition is the main problem, rates of obesity are also increasing, so that while many in the population suffer from the disease of hunger, many others are suffering from the problems of overnutrition. Globally the ratio of overweight: underfed people is 1.4:1. In developed countries this ratio is 11.8:1, and in developing countries it is 0.7:1.

The causes of obesity

The three-fold increase in obesity in less that a quarter of a century cannot be the result of genetic change in the population. Rather, it is the result of increased availability and consumption of food, coupled with decreased physical activity.

In most countries, the amount of food available per head of population has increased over the last three to four decades. Of course, this does not take account of wastage, which may be a considerable proportion of food that is purchased. At the same time, the cost of food has decreased in real terms in most developed countries—people have to spend a smaller percentage of their income on food than half a century ago. Perhaps more importantly, the consumption of supermarket prepared meals and food from fast food restaurants has increased, and many of these foods are high in fat and sugar, yielding more calories per serving than many home-prepared foods. It is therefore very easy to over eat and to have an excessive calorie intake. One calculation suggests that in the USA the percentage of food spending on meals outside the home increased from 30 to 40 per cent between the 1970s and 2000, but the percentage of calories consumed outside the home increased from 15 to 38 per cent over the same period.

The other factor in obesity is low energy expenditure. The average physical activity level (PAL) of adults in UK is only 1.4 x Basal Metabolic Rate (BMR). A desirable PAL for fitness is 1.7 x BMR, and this is achieved by only 22 per cent of men and 13 per cent of women.

Physical activity has decreased considerably over the last half century, for a number of reasons. Most leisure activities now involve spectator sports rather than playing on the field—and more people watch sport from armchairs in front of television sets than in the stands at the sports venue. Perhaps more worryingly, children spend more leisure time with computers and games consoles than playing outdoors. One study has linked an increase in rickets among adolescents to such indoor activities.

Most people now walk less and use cars or public transport more. Either because of laziness or because of real or perceived fears about safety, most children are now driven to school rather than being allowed to walk. Many people will wait for several minutes to take a lift for one or two flights of stairs rather than performing even this moderate exercise.

At the same time, with some very obvious exceptions, most work is now less physically demanding than it was half a century ago. There is increased mechanization in factories, more jobs are sedentary, with less need to walk around an office or factory. Automated washing machines need far less effort than doing laundry by hand; powered hedge trimmers and lawn mowers reduce the physical exertion of gardening.

How can overweight people lose weight?

There is an apparently simple answer to this question—eat less and exercise more. The increase in obesity tells us that the solution is not so simple. In fact, there are two separate but related problems: to reduce weight to within the desirable range; and to maintain that desirable weight afterwards.

There are many diets and slimming regimes that will allow someone to lose weight—if they follow the diet correctly. Long-term maintenance is more of a problem, and many of the popular weight reducing diets do not educate people in how to eat sensibly after they have achieved their target weight. The diet for maintenance of desirable weight is the same as the prudent diet discussed in Chapter 5: a total energy intake to permit maintenance of body weight, with 30 per cent of energy from fat, and only one-third of that fat as saturated fat, and 55 per cent of energy from carbohydrates (mainly as starches, with only 10 per cent of energy from sugars).

Adipose tissue contains about 15 per cent water, 5 per cent protein, and 80 per cent fat. This means that a gram of adipose tissue yields 7.4 kcal. We can calculate from this that a deficit of 500 kcal per day will lead to utilization of 68g of adipose tissue per day, or 476g in a week. If we assume a total energy expenditure (and therefore requirement) of 2,500 kcal/day, then even with total starvation the maximum possible weight loss will be 2.4kg (5 lb 5 oz) per week. It is important to bear this in mind when evaluating the claims for weight loss that are made for some diets. While the initial rate of weight loss as food intake is reduced may be higher in the first week, as a result of losing the water that is associated with tissue reserves of carbohydrates, after this even total starvation will only give a loss of 2.4kg (5 lb 5 oz)/week.

It is relatively easy for a dietitian to formulate a diet for weight reduction, by measuring or estimating the patient's current energy intake, then reducing it by about 10–20 per cent until the target weight has been achieved. It is less easy for someone to formulate his or her own weight reducing diet without having recourse to tables of food composition and performing relatively complex calculations. Labelling of foods with energy yield and fat and sugar content helps, but it is still tedious, and there are ways of making life easier for the would-be slimmer.

Prescriptive menus. Many obese people have relatively poor appetite control and are helped by having very prescriptive menus—with little or no choice of what to eat at each meal, and no choice of how much to eat. A number of companies now make this easy for the dieter by providing precisely formulated pre-prepared meals, either available from supermarkets or delivered to the home.

Traffic light lists of foods. A simple way of reducing energy intake is to have three lists of foods, which are coded like traffic lights. Red means high calorie foods, and foods high in fat and sugars, which should be eaten only in small amounts. Amber means foods that can be eaten in relatively larger amounts, but still with caution. Green means foods than can be eaten (within reason) in unlimited amounts—especially vegetables and other foods that are high in water and low in calories.

Exchange lists and 'points'. An alternative, which allows considerably more choice than prescriptive menus, but requires more discipline than traffic light lists, is to have lists of foods that are interchangeable, or have 'points', based on calorie and fat content. The dieter can now choose what to eat, as long as s/he keeps to the total number of points allowed each day. Of course, it is possible to formulate a very inadequate and inappropriate diet this way, for example by swapping all the points allowed for servings of meat and fish to points from chocolates, biscuits, and cakes.

High fibre diets. Diets that are rich in fruits and vegetables and whole grain cereals are high in dietary fibre, which is not digested and has very low energy yield. However, a high fibre diet will promote a feeling of fullness—many people complain that they feel hungry on slimming diets that are low in fibre.

Very low calorie diets and meal replacements. Consuming no more than 500 kcal/day will certainly permit a good rate of weight loss, and a number of diets achieve this by providing nutrient-rich low-calorie preparations to be eaten or drunk in place of one or more meals each day. However, once the target weight has been reached, the slimmer has not learnt any new eating habits, and is likely to revert to high calorie foods and regain the lost weight.

Very low carbohydrate diets. Very low carbohydrate diets, allowing more or less unlimited fat and protein, do work for weight reduction. This is partly because on a very low carbohydrate diet you become ketotic (producing large amounts of ketone bodies as a fuel for muscle), leading to nausea and loss of appetite. In addition, there is a need to maintain an appropriate level of blood glucose for the brain, and this can be provided by synthesizing glucose from the amino acids provided by protein. This is an energy expensive process, so it increases the utilization of body fat reserves to provide the energy needed.

Help and support. Many general practices now have a dietitian who can not only help people to formulate a diet, but can also arrange for regular meetings to assess their progress. However, this is extremely expensive, either for the patient or for the health service. An alternative, which has great success, is provided by slimming clubs of one kind or another. Typically, you receive appropriate dietary advice and are set a target weight as well as a time in which to achieve it. In return for a modest fee, there are weekly meetings at which you are weighed, and can discuss any problems with fellow slimmers and group leaders. Group leaders are typically people who have successfully lost weight (and maintained a desirable weight) on the same programme, and who therefore know all the problems of compliance that you are likely to encounter.

Sweeteners and fat replacers. For people with a sweet tooth, there are a number of non-caloric sweeteners available. Some are only suitable as 'table top' sweeteners to be used in tea, coffee, and low calorie soft drinks; others can be used in cooking to make cakes and desserts, or jams.

Many traditional foods that are high in fat are available as low fat alternatives, such as skimmed milk, low fat cheeses and sausages, as well as spreads to replace butter or margarine, containing only 40–50 per cent fat, and sometimes less—compared with 80 per cent fat in butter or margarine.

There are fat replacers based on protein and carbohydrate that have the same texture in the mouth as fat and can be used in some manufactured foods. Other fat replacers are based on compounds of fatty acids with sucrose; these are not digested at all, so have zero energy yield, but can be used for frying or baking.

Drugs to aid weight loss. Over the years a number of drugs have been developed to aid weight loss. Some of these acted by increasing the metabolic rate so that energy expenditure was increased. The result of this was a low grade fever—hardly a pleasant way of losing weight.

Slimming patches purport to contain iodine from seaweed, although in at least some cases there is no iodine present, because iodine is volatile. The theory behind their use is that if you are iodine deficient you produce little thyroid hormone, your metabolic rate falls, and so that you become overweight and lethargic. This is true, as is the fact that people who over-produce thyroid hormone because of thyroid disease have a high metabolic rate, lose weight, and are thin. However, if you are not iodine deficient and do not have thyroid disease, providing additional iodine does not increase metabolic rate and does not help weight loss.

A number of drugs have been developed to suppress appetite by acting on the appetite control centres of the brain. While they are successful, most of them are potentially or actually addictive, and some have serious side-effects. Many appetite suppressant drugs have now been withdrawn, although some are still available on prescription, and some are available by online purchase (but there is no guarantee of quality or safety with drugs bought online).

Drugs to inhibit carbohydrate digestion have some efficacy, and drugs to inhibit fat digestion are certainly effective, although they have the side effect of causing foul smelling, fatty diarrhoea if you continue to consume a relatively large amount of fat.

Surgery for obesity. It was noted above that obese people are considerably more at risk during surgery than lean people. Any surgical intervention to remove a significant part of the intestinal tract or part of the stomach is irreversible. This means that surgery must be considered as being the last resort—for the obese person who has genuinely tried to lose weight by other means.

Diets that (probably) will not work. There is a never-ending list of diets that are unlikely to be successful. Some are based on misconceptions, others are based on a very limited list of foods, with the idea that you will become bored and eat very little. Such diets (e.g. the cabbage diet, based on eating little apart from cabbage soup; diets based on mango and fresh pineapple; etc.) are obviously unbalanced and nutritionally unsound. Fortunately, most people become bored with the limitations of the diet before they develop severe nutritional deficiencies.

Food combining (sometimes called the Hay diet) is based on the concept of not eating protein and carbohydrate at the same meal—but this ignores the fact that almost all carbohydrate containing foods also contain significant amounts of protein.

The macrobiotic diet is a system of eating associated with Zen Buddhism. It consists of several stages, finally reaching Diet 7, which is restricted to cereals. Cases of severe malnutrition have been reported on this diet. It involves the Chinese concept of yin (female) and yang (male), whereby foods, and even different vitamins (indeed, everything in life), are predominantly one or the other, and must be balanced.

The pH diet is based on balancing the intake of acid forming and base forming foods, with little or no scientific basis, and the zone diet on the unfounded belief that each meal should comprise a fixed proportion of macronutrients: 40 per cent carbohydrate, 30 per cent fat, and 30 per cent protein.

Detox diets are based on the unfounded belief that toxins from food accumulate in the body, slowing metabolism and leading to weight gain. There is no evidence for this. A period of fasting and strict avoidance of such supposed toxins as caffeine and food additives is claimed to be beneficial. Various herbal supplements are often included in 'detox diets', with little or no evidence of efficacy. Proponents claim that the sensation of lightheadedness that occurs after a few days of more or less complete fasting is the result of toxins being released, while in fact it is the result of low blood glucose and ketosis—as a result of starvation.

Chapter 5
Diet and health

Patterns of disease and mortality differ around the world, and one of the factors that can be correlated with many of the differences is diet, although there are obviously other environmental (and genetic) factors involved. This chapter is concerned with the ways in which we can gather evidence that diet is, or may be, a factor in the development of chronic non-communicable diseases (especially atherosclerosis, coronary heart disease, hypertension (high blood pressure), and cancer), and how we can use these findings to produce guidelines for a prudent diet and to promote healthy eating.

At one time these chronic non-communicable diseases were known as diseases of affluence, because they were seen mainly in affluent Western countries and mainly among the wealthier sections of society. Increasingly, however, they are becoming major causes of premature death in developing countries, and are more common among the poorer, rather than wealthier, sections of society in developed countries.

The relative amounts of fat, carbohydrate, and protein in the diet are important, as is the mixture of different types of carbohydrate and fat. Consumption of alcohol may have both beneficial and adverse effects on health. A wide variety of compounds in foods (and especially in fruits and vegetables) may also have beneficial effects.

How we gather evidence linking diet and health

Different types of epidemiological study can give information about diet and health. The first clues often come from looking at changes in diet over the past 100 or so years, coupled with changes in the pattern of disease. Such studies suggest that, in parallel with the increase in atherosclerosis, cardiovascular disease, and cancer, there have been increases in the total amount of fat and sugar consumed, with a reduction in starch and dietary fibre. A considerably greater proportion of the fat consumed is animal fat, which is largely saturated. One obvious problem with this comparison is that people now live longer now than they did 100 years ago. This is partly because the diseases associated with under-nutrition are now rare in developed countries, and partly because many infectious diseases that were common killers can now be treated with antibiotics and anti-viral drugs. The provision of clean drinking water and effective management of sewage have also been important factors.

A great deal can be learnt from studying people who have migrated from one country to another, and comparing their patterns of disease, and their diets, with relatives who have remained in the mother country. Similarly, we can look at patterns of disease in different countries—for example, there is a 100-fold difference in the incidence of breast and prostate cancer between West Africa and the USA. Are there any differences in diet that might explain this? Vegetables form a large part of the traditional Japanese and Chinese diets, as does fish in Japan and near the coast in China. The oestrogen-like compounds in soya products may explain the lower incidence of breast and prostate cancer in China and Japan compared with that in Western countries. The traditional Mediterranean diet, rich in fruits and vegetables, with more fish and seafood than meat, and moderate wine consumption is associated with considerably lower incidence of cardiovascular disease than Northern Europe.

Many studies have shown that there is a significant international correlation between fat intake and breast cancer. Such studies assume that the data on food availability in different countries are comparable. The main problem here is that diet is only one of many factors that differ between different countries, and many other lifestyle and environmental factors may also be important. More detailed international correlation studies involve taking blood samples for laboratory studies. The Seven Countries study, which started in the 1950s and has continued to the present, first established that elevated serum cholesterol was a major factor in atherosclerosis and coronary heart disease.

At a more individual level, we can look at people with a given disease and compare them with people who are free from the disease, but matched for age, sex, lifestyle, and as many other factors as possible. This is a case-control study. It gives better information than international correlation studies, and in many studies we also have information not only on diet but also on results from laboratory tests to measure individual nutrients and markers of nutritional status in blood and urine samples.

The problem with case-control studies is that we are looking at people who already have the disease, but the initiation of cancer or cardiovascular disease occurs many years before the disease becomes apparent. What we really need to know is what these people were eating 10 to 20 years ago. Equally, the disease itself may affect the metabolism of nutrients. These problems can be overcome with long-term prospective studies, in which people are followed for many years, with records of diet and other lifestyle factors at the beginning and at frequent intervals throughout the study. Many such studies also include laboratory tests, physical examination, and questionnaires at intervals. The oldest such study is the 1946 birth cohort study in the UK. Every child born in the second week of March 1946 is still being followed, and new cohorts have been added. Other prospective studies include the Framingham study in the USA, which has followed everyone in the town since 1948; the Nurses' Health Study (again in the USA) which has followed over 100,000 nurses since 1976; the Whitehall Study, in which civil servants in England have been followed since 1967; and the European Prospective Investigation into Cancer and Nutrition (EPIC), which has followed half a million people in ten European countries since the 1990s.

Experimental studies can also give useful information. Once it had been established that elevated serum cholesterol was a risk factor for atherosclerosis and coronary heart disease, and epidemiological studies suggested that different types of fat may affect serum cholesterol differently, a series of experiments was

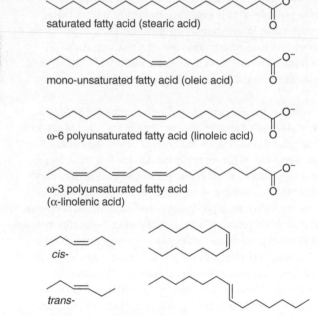

saturated fatty acid (stearic acid)

mono-unsaturated fatty acid (oleic acid)

ω-6 polyunsaturated fatty acid (linoleic acid)

ω-3 polyunsaturated fatty acid
(α-linolenic acid)

cis-

trans-

1. Saturated and unsaturated fatty acids, and the *cis-* and *trans-* arrangements around a double bond

conducted in the 1960s. People were fed standardized diets in which the total amount of fat remained constant, but where mono-unsaturated fat was replaced with either saturated or polyunsaturated fat (see Figure 1). The amount of cholesterol in the diets was also varied in separate experiments. The results showed that compared with mono-unsaturated fat, saturated fats increase serum cholesterol proportionally to twice the intake, while polyunsaturated fats decrease it proportionally with intake. Dietary cholesterol also increases serum cholesterol, but only proportionally to the square root of intake.

Other studies have investigated the effects of changes in diet on blood pressure, and have identified a high salt intake and excessive alcohol consumption as significant risk factors. There have also been trials of supplements of individual nutrients to reduce the risk of developing cancer.

Guidelines for a prudent diet

These epidemiological and experimental studies have provided evidence for a dietary pattern that is associated with reduced risk of developing cancer, atherosclerosis and cardiovascular disease, hypertension and stroke, and type II diabetes. As discussed earlier, such a diet provides 30 per cent of energy from fat (with only about 30 per cent of this fat being saturated and 6 to 10 per cent being polyunsaturated fat; see Figure 1 for the structures of the different types of fatty acids in dietary fats); 55 per cent of energy from carbohydrates (mainly starch, with only 10 per cent of energy from sugars); and 15 per cent of energy from protein.

Table 5 compares this prudent diet with the average Western diet—where there is a need to reduce total fat and sugar consumption, and to increase starch consumption. At the same time, the proportion of fat that is saturated needs to be reduced; average intakes of mono- and polyunsaturated fats are about right, so that all of the reduction in fat intake should be achieved by

Table 5. Guidelines for percentage of energy from fats, carbohydrates, and proteins in a prudent diet compared with average Western diets

	Western average (%)	Desirable (%)
Total fat	40	30
saturated fatty acids	17	10
mono-unsaturated fatty acids	12	12
polyunsaturated fatty acids	6	6
trans-fatty acids	2–3	<1
Total carbohydrate	43	55
free sugars	Variable	10
Protein	14–15	14–15

From data reported by WHO (1990). *Diet, Nutrition and the Prevention of Chronic Diseases.* WHO Technical Reports Series 797, Geneva reducing saturated fat intake. Average salt intake is considerably in excess of requirements, and should be reduced to minimize the risk of hypertension. Average intakes of alcohol are also greater than is considered desirable for good health.

Polyunsaturated fatty acids. Polyunsaturated fatty acids are those with two or more double bonds in the molecule (see Figure 1). They are important in the structure of cell membranes, and are the precursors of prostaglandins and related compounds that have hormone-like actions. Enzymes in the body are capable of increasing the chain length of polyunsaturated fatty acids up to the 20 carbons that are required for prostaglandin synthesis, and of introducing additional double bonds between an existing double bond and the carboxyl group of the fatty acid. However, there are no human enzymes that are capable of introducing additional double bonds between the terminal methyl group and the first existing double bond. As shown in Figure 1, there are two families of polyunsaturated fatty acids, ω3 (omega-3) and ω6 (omega-6), that give rise to different families of prostaglandins and related compounds, with different actions in the body. Since it is not possible to convert a ω6 fatty acid to a ω3 fatty acid, there is a need for both in the diet. The ratio of ω3 to ω6 in the diet is important, because the same enzymes are involved in metabolizing both families of polyunsaturated fatty acids, and they compete with each other. The major dietary sources of ω6 polyunsaturated fatty acids are plant oils, and the major sources of ω3 fatty acids are oily fish such as salmon, trout, and herring, as well as fish liver oils. Fish oils provide ready-formed long-chain ω3 fatty acids and there is good evidence that eating one or two servings of oily fish a week has health benefits and reduces the chances of cardiovascular disease.

Trans-fats. Most of the naturally occurring unsaturated fatty acids have the *cis*-conformation—as shown in Figure 1, the chain of carbon atoms continues on the same side of the double bond. When liquid oils are treated to convert some of the unsaturated fatty acids to saturated fatty acids for the manufacture of spreads and other solid fats that can be used for food manufacture, some of the unsaturated fatty acids undergo a change from the *cis*-conformation to the *trans*-conformation. Evidence has accumulated over the past few years that not only do these *trans*-fatty acids not have the same beneficial effects as *cis*-unsaturated fatty acids, but they are actually more hazardous to health than saturated fatty acids. *Trans*-fatty acids should provide no more than 1 per cent of energy intake. Many food manufacturers have eliminated *trans*-fatty acids from their products, by using alternative, but more expensive, methods of preparing solid fats from liquid oils.

Dietary fibre. Plant cell walls contain a variety of compounds that are not digested, but nevertheless have an important role in the diet. Collectively these compounds are referred to as dietary fibre or non-starch polysaccharides. The term 'dietary fibre' is misleading in that few of the compounds involved actually form fibres, and indeed some (the plant gums) are soluble, but undigested, carbohydrates. It is more correct to call them non-starch polysaccharides. All plant foods contain dietary fibre in varying amounts. Whole grain cereals are an especially rich source, but much is lost when wheat is refined to produce white flour.

At the simplest level, dietary fibre provides bulk in the diet. This permits easier passage of food through the gut and reduces the risk of either constipation or diarrhoea. A low fibre diet is associated with increased risk of diverticular disease of the colon and haemorrhoids, and increasing fibre intake helps to relieve both conditions.

Dietary fibre also physically adsorbs a number of compounds in the diet that are potentially liable to cause cancer, so preventing their absorption. It also adsorbs bile salts, which are secreted from the gall bladder into the intestine for fat digestion and absorption.

This means that less of the secreted bile salts is re-absorbed, so that there has to be more synthesis in the liver. The precursor for bile salt synthesis is cholesterol, so an increased intake of dietary fibre helps to lower serum cholesterol.

The plant gums and other compounds that make up soluble dietary fibre slow the rate of absorption of nutrients from the gut. This is beneficial for people with diabetes, since the main cause of problems of controlling blood glucose arise when there is a rapid increase in glucose becoming available after a meal. A number of studies have shown that consuming a supplement of soluble dietary fibre before a meal improves control of blood glucose.

Although we cannot digest the various compounds that make up dietary fibre, they do provide a substrate for intestinal bacteria, which can ferment them. This helps to maintain a healthy population of intestinal bacteria, which can compete with pathogenic bacteria that cause food poisoning. Some of the products of this bacterial fermentation are also available to the cells lining the intestinal tract. They provide a major metabolic fuel for these cells, and there is some evidence that they protect against the development of cancer of the colon.

Fruits and vegetables—five servings a day. All of the epidemiological evidence suggests that people who consume an average of five servings of fruit and vegetables a day are less at risk of obesity, cardiovascular disease, and cancer. It does not matter if these are fresh, frozen, or canned, and fruit juices are also beneficial, although they may provide undesirably high levels of soluble sugars that can cause dental decay. The benefits of fruit and vegetable consumption are partly due to the beneficial effects of dietary fibre discussed above, and partly to the fact that a diet that is rich in fruit and vegetables will be relatively low in fat, and especially saturated fat. A relatively high fibre diet is beneficial for weight reduction because it helps to prevent feelings of emptiness and hunger while providing relatively few calories. In addition, fruits and vegetables provide a good source of vitamins and minerals, as well as a large number of other compounds that, while not dietary essentials, have a protective effect against cancer and cardiovascular disease.

Alcohol. Most countries have guidelines on prudent levels of alcohol consumption. In the UK, the Royal College of Physicians first developed guidelines for alcohol consumption in the 1990s. They defined a unit of alcohol as being equivalent to 8g of pure alcohol—this is the amount in half pint of beer, 100 ml of wine (a small glass), or a single 25 ml measure of spirits. The prudent upper level of consumption is 21 units per week for men and 14 units per week for women. The sex difference is because the liver, which is where alcohol is metabolized, is smaller in women than in men, so that women are more at risk from the adverse effects of excessive alcohol consumption than are men. The UK Department of Health modified these guidelines in 1995, setting the prudent upper limit as 4 units per day for men and 3 units per day for women. This was not intended to increase the upper level of alcohol intake, but rather to emphasize the point that binge drinking (consuming the whole week's 'allowance' in one evening) is more hazardous to health than regular consumption of moderate amounts.

Free radicals and antioxidants. One of the theories to explain the underlying cause of cancer and atherosclerosis is that tissues are damaged by free radicals. Free radicals are highly reactive molecules that have an unpaired electron. When a radical collides with another molecule, it becomes stable by removing or donating a single electron, but in the process it generates a new radical. Radicals can cause damage to DNA, leading to possible mutations and the development of cancer; and to fats, leading to the development of atherosclerosis; as well as to proteins, leading to the development of auto-immune diseases, including rheumatoid arthritis. The radicals that cause the most damage are oxygen radicals, and compounds that provide protection against radical damage are generally referred to as antioxidants.

Oxygen radicals are formed in the body as part of normal metabolism and protection against infection; it is estimated that about 5 per cent of the oxygen we consume each day forms potentially damaging radicals. Many epidemiological studies have shown that relatively high blood concentrations of antioxidants such as β-carotene and vitamins C and E are associated with lower risk of cancer and cardiovascular disease. However, intervention trials with high doses of antioxidants have not shown the expected protection, and many of the trials of β-carotene and vitamin E have shown increased mortality among those taking the supposedly protective supplements.

There are three possible explanations for this adverse effect of high dose antioxidant supplements. Antioxidants act by forming stable radicals that persist long enough to penetrate deeper into tissues, so causing more damage. Some antioxidants, especially β-carotene, may act as antioxidants in tissues where there is little free oxygen, but in tissues such as the lung they become pro-oxidants, generating damaging oxygen radicals. The Food Standards Agency in UK has warned smokers not to take β-carotene supplements because of the increased risk of lung cancer. Perhaps most importantly, antioxidants may also have an adverse effect because much of the signalling for damaged cells that might go on to develop into cancers to undergo programmed cell death depends on oxygen radicals. High concentrations of antioxidants will quench these important signalling radicals, leading to survival of potentially cancerous cells.

Publicizing healthy eating

There are two main approaches to publicizing the key messages about healthy eating and a prudent diet: nutritional labelling of foods and public health campaigns that translate the nutritional guidelines in Table 5 into foods.

Nutritional labelling of packaged and manufactured foods provides a great deal of information: the energy yield, fat (and saturated fat), carbohydrate (and sugars), and vitamin and mineral content, both as amount per serving or per 100g and also as percentage of the reference intake, daily value, or guideline daily amount. Increasingly, in addition to nutritional labelling, manufacturers are being encouraged (and in some countries required) to have 'front of package' labelling that highlights the fat, saturated fat, sugar, and salt content of the food. This may take the form of a 'traffic light' colour coded label—green for low fat, saturated fat, sugar, and salt; amber for medium; and red for high. Alternatively, labels show the energy, fat, saturated fat, sugar, and salt content as the amount and as a percentage of the guideline daily amount or daily value—the amount called for by the prudent diet discussed above. The most successful front of package labels use both schemes—traffic lights plus the amount and percentage of guideline daily amount.

While such labelling helps the discriminating consumer to make healthy choices, it is relatively little help in converting nutritional guidelines into foods. The food pyramid (see Figure 2) has the starchy foods that should provide the main part of the diet at the base, with fruit and vegetables in the next row, then dairy produce, meat, and fish, and with foods that should be eaten sparingly (fats, oils, and sweets) at the apex. Apart from fats, oils, and sweets, there is a suggestion of how many servings of each group of foods should be consumed each day. The food pyramid has been criticized for the fact that the foods that should be eaten in smallest amount are shown at the top of the pyramid, which implies to some people that they are the most important foods.

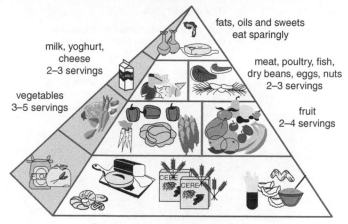

bread, cereals, rice and pasta 6–11 servings

2. The food pyramid

In the UK, the Foods Standards Agency has developed the 'eatwell plate' (formerly called the balanced plate) shown in Figure 3. Here the five groups of foods (fruit and vegetables, bread, cereals and potatoes, meat, fish and alternatives, milk and dairy foods, and foods and drinks containing fat and sugar), are shown as sectors of the plate representing the relative amounts that should be eaten each day. The USA has abandoned the food pyramid and now uses a simple four sector plate ('choose my plate' in Figure 3) for fruit, vegetables (half the plate is fruit and vegetables), grains (more than a quarter of the plate), and protein—with a separate container for dairy produce. There is no mention of fats, oils, and sugars that should be consumed in limited amounts, since the aim is to emphasize a positive message.

(a)

The eatwell plate

Use the eatwell plate to help you get the balance right. It shows how much of what you eat should come from each food group.

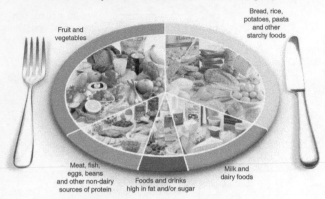

Fruit and vegetables

Bread, rice, potatoes, pasta and other starchy foods

Meat, fish, eggs, beans and other non-dairy sources of protein

Foods and drinks high in fat and/or sugar

Milk and dairy foods

Public Health England in association with the Welsh Government, the Scottish Government, and the Food Standards Agency in Northern Ireland

(b)

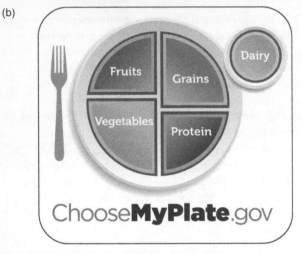

3. a) The 'eatwell plate' and b) 'choose my plate'

62

Chapter 6
Under-nutrition

Severe under-nutrition is generally associated with developing countries where food is in short supply, affecting some 162 million people worldwide. In India, 40 per cent of the population is underweight, and a further 10 per cent is severely malnourished. In sub-Saharan Africa, 10 to 20 per cent of the population of different countries is underweight. Even in developed countries, about 2 per cent of the population (a total of 11 million people world-wide) is significantly undernourished, and can be classified as having moderate protein-energy malnutrition.

Three conditions are classified as protein-energy malnutrition: marasmus, which affects adults and children; kwashiorkor, which affects young children; and cachexia, which is associated with advanced cancer and other chronic diseases, and involves increased metabolic rate as well as reduced food intake.

The term protein-energy malnutrition does not imply that there is a deficit of protein per se, rather that there is a lack of food, so that much of the dietary protein is being used as a metabolic fuel rather than for tissue protein synthesis. A body mass index (BMI) between 17 and 18.4 is classified as moderate, 16 to 17 as moderately severe, and less that 16 as severe protein-energy malnutrition. BMI between 18.5 and 20 is considered to be underweight, but is not associated with any adverse outcomes.

Through the last quarter of the 20th century there was an increase in food availability in almost all countries, largely as a result of increased yields of staple cereals, due to the 'green revolution'. Since then the condition has worsened in many countries, for a variety of reasons. Droughts, floods, and wars have led to considerable losses of crops, and what should be food crops such as maize and soya are increasingly used to produce biofuels to replace oil. There is increasing loss of agricultural land by desertification in sub-Saharan Africa and elsewhere. At the same time, the world population has increased from 5 billion in 1997 to 7 billion in 2010, and is predicted to increase to 11 billion by the end of the 21st century. Finally, increasing affluence in fast developing countries such as China, India, and Brazil has led to demands for a more Western style of diet, with more meat and less reliance on cereals and root crops as the dietary staples. This means that more of the cereals, legumes, and root crops are used to feed livestock. Although the animals are eaten by human beings, this is considerably less efficient in terms of utilization of the crops than if they were eaten directly.

Marasmus

The name 'marasmus' comes from the Greek for wasting, and this is the most obvious feature of the severely underfed person—severe wasting of muscle with negligible fat reserves. The condition is the predictable outcome of a prolonged inadequate intake of food. Adipose tissue reserves of fat are used as the main metabolic fuel, but there is a need to maintain a supply of glucose for the brain, by use of amino acids from protein turnover for synthesis of glucose. The rate of tissue protein breakdown continues at a more or less normal rate, but replacement synthesis is severely reduced, both because of the use of amino acids for glucose synthesis and also because of the high energy cost of protein synthesis. Once adipose tissue reserves are more or less exhausted, there is a considerable increase in the rate of protein loss, and eventually essential tissue proteins are lost, leading to death.

The reduced rate of protein synthesis leads to impaired immune system responses, so that resistance to infection is low, and what might be considered to be a mild infection may be fatal. There is also a reduction in the rate of tissue cell proliferation. This especially affects cells in the gastro-intestinal tract, which turn over rapidly. As a result there is considerable flattening of the intestinal villi (the finger-like projections of the intestinal wall where most nutrients are absorbed) and loss of the normal absorptive area in the gut. This leads to diarrhoea and failure to absorb much of such food as is available.

Cachexia

'Cachexia' comes from the Greek for 'in a bad state or condition'. Superficially, this condition resembles marasmus, in that the patient is severely emaciated, with negligible fat reserves and considerable muscle loss. The condition is seen in patients with advanced cancer, AIDS, tuberculosis, and chronic heart and lung disease.

To some extent the condition can be attributed to reduced food intake—the patient's appetite may be poor because of illness, and many of the drugs used cause nausea (so reducing appetite) or distort the senses of taste and smell, so that many foods become aversive. At the same time, many of the drugs used in cancer chemotherapy inhibit cell division, so that there is flattening of the villi in the small intestine that normally provide the large surface area for absorption of nutrients. This leads to failure to absorb nutrients.

There are two differences between marasmus and cachexia: the cachetic patient has a high metabolic rate, and in addition to reduced protein synthesis there is an increased rate of protein breakdown. Both are responses to hormones and other factors produced either by the body in response to the disease or, in the case of cancer, to factors produced by the tumours. The increased metabolic rate in cachexia leads to fever and an increased need for metabolic fuels, so hastening the development of malnutrition.

Kwashiorkor

Kwashiorkor was first described in Ghana in 1935, and the word is the Ga name for the disease affecting undernourished children. Traditionally it develops when the child is weaned (which may be as late as age 2 to 3 years), and the early hypothesis was that kwashiorkor developed because the child was fed on a starchy gruel with little or no protein. However, kwashiorkor is not the result of an adequate energy intake with inadequate protein, but the result of lack of food overall. Protein-deficient children show stunted growth, but children with kwashiorkor are less stunted than those with marasmus. Furthermore, the condition begins to resolve when the child is given an adequate supply of energy (often in the form of sugar solution), before the protein intake is increased.

Kwashiorkor is frequently precipitated in an undernourished child by an infection, and it is likely that the precipitating factor is tissue damage by radicals produced by white blood cells (macrophages) that are activated to fight the infection.

Kwashiorkor differs from marasmus in that there is considerable retention of fluid under the skin. This oedema masks the muscle wasting, so that the child with kwashiorkor may appear to be chubby. There is also fatty infiltration of the liver, leading to a pot belly. The child's hair is thin, wispy, and underpigmented, and the child has a characteristic miserable facial expression and a sunburn-like dermatitis.

A child who is 60 to 80 per cent of expected weight for age without oedema is considered to be undernourished; if there is also oedema, the problem is kwashiorkor. If the child is less than

60 per cent of expected weight for age without oedema, this is marasmus. If there is also oedema, this is marasmic kwashiorkor, which is the most serious condition. In emergency situations, it is children with marasmic kwashiorkor who have the first priority for treatment.

Malnutrition in developed countries

Even in developed countries, where obesity is the main cause for concern, a significant number of people are undernourished. In the UK, 5 per cent of adults have a BMI of less than 20, and 2 per cent below 18.5, which is moderate protein-energy malnutrition. Three per cent of older men and 6 per cent of women living in their own homes and looking after themselves are undernourished. For elderly people living in care homes, the situation is worse, with 16 per cent of men and 15 per cent of women significantly undernourished. One study showed that 40 per cent of consecutive patients admitted to hospital were undernourished, and two-thirds of those staying in hospital for more than a week lost weight, even those who were undernourished on admission. The cost to the National Health Service of treating the consequences of malnutrition in UK is estimated at around £7 billion a year—almost twice the cost of treating the consequences of obesity.

Malnutrition leads to impaired immune responses, predisposing the individual to infection. The loss of muscle may result in increased fatiguability, inability to work, and falls. Inactivity as a result of loss of muscle predisposes individuals to blood clots and also leads to further muscle loss. Loss of respiratory muscle strength leads to poor cough pressure, which creates a predisposition to chest infections, poor recovery from chest infections, and increased risk under general anaesthesia. The healing of wounds is impaired, and recovery from illness is prolonged, leading to an increased length of stay in hospital and delayed return to work.

Even when not accompanied by physical illness, malnutrition leads to apathy, depression, self-neglect, loss of libido, and deterioration in social interactions.

The most vulnerable sections of the population are those living at or below the poverty line; those who are outside the welfare net for one reason or another; and the bereaved elderly, who may have little motivation to cook and eat. There are also problems in care homes and hospitals.

Chapter 7
Vitamins and minerals

In addition to sources of energy and protein, there is a need for two further groups of nutrients in the diet, in relatively small amounts: mineral salts and vitamins. Together these are known as micronutrients, because they are required in small amounts.

The vitamins were discovered at the beginning of the 20th century as a group of organic compounds (and hence distinct from essential minerals) that are required in the diet in small amounts (milligrams or micrograms per day), and so distinct from the essential amino acids that are required in gram amounts. They are essential for maintenance of normal health, growth, and metabolic integrity. Deficiency leads to more or less specific clinical signs and symptoms and metabolic disturbances, and replacing the vitamin in the diet will prevent or cure the deficiency disease. Vitamins cannot be made in the body and must be provided in the diet. There are two exceptions here. Vitamin D can be synthesized in the skin if there is adequate sunlight exposure, and niacin can be synthesized from the essential amino acid tryptophan. However, deficiencies of both do occur.

There is another group of compounds found mainly in plants that are not dietary essentials, but may be beneficial. Collectively these are known as phytonutrients. They have a number of different potentially protective actions against cancer and cardiovascular disease.

Essential minerals

Two minerals, iron and calcium, are required in relatively large amounts. The remainder of minerals are required in small amounts and are sometimes called trace elements; some (ultra-trace elements) are required in very small amounts. Deficiency of the ultra-trace minerals is unlikely, but deficiency of other minerals does occur, especially where locally grown foods provide the main intake and the soil is deficient in a mineral. Deficiencies of iron and iodine are major problems of public health worldwide, and iron and iodine, together with vitamin A, are key micronutrient targets of the World Health Organization.

Table 6 shows the essential minerals classified by their functions in the body. Some minerals appear more than once—for example, calcium is important in the structure of bone, but also has an important role in responses to hormones.

Iron. The greatest need for iron in the body is for synthesis of the protein haemoglobin, which transports oxygen in red blood cells. It is also required for the oxygen transport protein myoglobin in muscle, and in a large number of enzymes. Iron deficiency is seen as anaemia—small, underpigmented red blood cells with a reduced capacity to transport oxygen. This leads to easy fatigue and breathlessness during exercise. It is especially a problem of women of child-bearing age, since losses of iron through menstrual blood loss are frequently greater than can be replaced from the diet. Worldwide, more than two billion people are iron deficient.

There are two sources of iron in the diet: haem from myoglobin in meat, and inorganic iron salts, mainly from plant foods. Iron absorption from the diet is poor, especially for inorganic iron salts;

Table 6. Minerals classified by their functions in the body

Functions	Mineral name
Structural function	calcium, magnesium, phosphate
Involved in membrane function	sodium, potassium
Function as prosthetic groups in enzymes	cobalt, copper, iron, molybdenum, selenium, zinc
Have a regulatory role or a role in hormone action	calcium, chromium, iodine, magnesium, manganese, sodium, potassium
Known to be essential, but whose function is unknown	silicon, vanadium, nickel, tin
Have effects in the body but are not considered to be essential	fluoride, lithium
May occur in foods, have no known function in the body and are known to be toxic in excess	aluminium, arsenic, antimony, boron, bromine, cadmium, caesium, germanium, lead, mercury, silver, strontium

the absorption of iron from haem is higher. However, the absorption of both is controlled, largely in response to the body's need for iron. There is no mechanism for excretion of excess iron that has been absorbed, and people with genetic defects in the regulation of iron absorption suffer from haemochromatosis—iron overload. This is characterized by bronze colouration of the skin, depletion of vitamin C, and damage to various tissues, including the pancreas, leading to the development of diabetes, as well as inflammation of joints and heart disease. Up to 10 per cent of the population is genetically at risk of iron overload if intake of iron is too high.

Inorganic iron in the diet must be chemically reduced before it can be absorbed into the cells of the small intestine, and it has been known for many years that when iron supplements are given for treatment of anaemia, they should be accompanied by vitamin C as a reducing agent, or taken with orange juice as a source of vitamin C, to improve absorption. Alcohol and meat protein also increase the absorption of inorganic iron. A number of dietary factors decrease the absorption of inorganic iron, including calcium, dietary fibre, tannins, and egg and soya proteins.

Once inside the intestinal cell, whether it is absorbed as inorganic iron or released from haem, iron is bound to a storage protein, ferritin. It is then transported into the bloodstream only if there is free transferrin available, without iron bound. Transferrin is the protein that transports iron to tissues that require it. If all the transferrin in the blood has iron bound (indicating that body iron reserves are adequate), iron cannot be transported out of the mucosal cells, and is lost in the faeces when the cells are shed. There is a further control over iron absorption. Transport from the intestinal cell onto transferrin requires the protein ferroportin, and ferroportin synthesis is regulated by a protein, hepcidin, which is synthesized in the liver in response to the state of body iron reserves.

Calcium. The body contains about 1kg of calcium, of which 99 per cent is in bones and teeth. There is thus obviously a need for an adequate intake of calcium for bone formation. Milk and dairy products are the main source of calcium in the diet, but cereals, fruits, and vegetables provide significant amounts. Calcium also has a role in regulating the activity of muscle, and in response to the actions of many hormones. The plasma concentration of calcium is tightly regulated. An excessively high plasma concentration of calcium can lead to calcification and hardening of soft tissues, including blood vessels. If the plasma concentration of calcium falls too low, neuro-muscular coordination is lost, leading to tetany and convulsions.

The absorption of calcium from the gut requires vitamin D, and in vitamin D deficiency there is not enough calcium available for normal formation of bone mineral. In children this leads to the disease of rickets, when bone that is formed as the child grows is soft and the long bones of the body bend. As they gradually become mineralized, so the bone remains deformed. The adult equivalent of rickets is osteomalacia. There is normal turnover of bone, with mobilization of mineral and erosion of bone proteins, followed by replacement bone synthesis. In calcium deficiency due to a lack of vitamin D there is insufficient calcium available to permit mineralization of this newly formed bone.

A normal consequence of ageing is loss of bone matrix proteins and calcium, leading to fragile, porous bones—the condition of osteoporosis. Osteoporotic bones fracture readily, in response to mild trauma, and when the condition affects the vertebrae there is serious curvature of the spine—so-called dowager's hump. Oestrogens and androgens stimulate the formation of new bone. Osteoporosis affects women more than men, because the loss of oestrogens at the menopause is abrupt while the loss of testosterone occurs more gradually, as men age.

There is some evidence that supplements of calcium and vitamin D in later life slow the progression of osteoporosis. However, the major factor affecting the rate of development of clinically significant osteoporosis is the peak density of the bones in early middle age. The denser the bones are to start with, the longer it will take for there to be enough bone loss to cause problems. This means that it is important to have an adequate intake of calcium (and vitamin D) from childhood through adolescence into middle age.

Iodine. Iodine is required for synthesis of the thyroid hormones, which control metabolic rate and the coordination of growth and development. In response to iodine deficiency, the thyroid gland in the neck enlarges in an attempt to synthesize enough of the hormones. In severe deficiency the enlarged gland may be as large as a football. This condition is iodine deficiency goitre. The thin, free-draining soils in inland upland areas over limestone are deficient in iodine. In many regions of the world, including the

Himalayas, the Matto Grosso of Brazil, and large areas of central Africa, the prevalence of iodine deficiency goitre was nearly 100 per cent before the introduction of preventative programmes. It was formerly a common problem in the Alps and in Derbyshire—indeed, at one time goitre was called 'Derbyshire neck'. Fish and other sea-foods are rich sources of iodine.

The iodine deficient goitrous patient has a low metabolic rate, gains weight, and has a dull mental apathy. Children born to iodine deficient mothers are very seriously affected, with deafness and severe mental impairment—the condition of goitrous cretinism.

In developed countries and urban areas of developing countries, the problem is prevented by provision of iodized salt, or the mandatory use of iodized salt for bread making. In less developed areas where this is not possible, medical teams give injections of iodized oil. An undesirable side-effect of improving iodine status in areas of deficiency is that adults whose thyroid glands have enlarged as a result of deficiency now become transiently hyperthyroid, as the enlarged gland synthesizes excessive amounts of thyroid hormones when iodine becomes available. However, this is considered to be an acceptable trade-off for preventing the severe effects of iodine deficiency in unborn and young children.

If iodine status is adequate, there is no evidence that any additional intake will cause hyperthyroidism unless the gland is enlarged as a result of previous deficiency. There is certainly no evidence that additional iodine will increase metabolic rate and aid weight loss.

Selenium. Selenium is required for synthesis of the amino acid selenocysteine, which is important in a number of enzymes, including glutathione peroxidase, which forms part of the antioxidant defences of the body, and the deiodinase enzyme that activates the thyroid hormone. Rich sources of selenium include Brazil nuts, fish and sea-foods, and organ meat (especially kidneys). Selenium deficiency is a problem in several areas of the world where the selenium content of the soil is low, including New Zealand, Finland, and large regions of China. Equally, there are regions of the world where the selenium content of the soil is so high that cattle cannot safely be grazed, and locally grown crops may contain undesirably high levels of selenium. There is concern in the UK that levels of selenium intake have fallen over the past quarter century, to the extent that average intakes are below requirements. This is largely because wheat that was formerly imported from Australia and North America (where soil selenium levels are relatively high) has been replaced by wheat grown in Europe (where soil selenium levels are relatively low).

There is a need to exercise caution with selenium supplements. A desirable level of intake is 55 μg/day, and once the activities of the various selenium-containing enzymes have been optimized, higher levels of intake have no additional effect. However, at intakes above about 400 μg/day, signs of selenium toxicity develop. In addition to loss of hair and nails, selenium poisoning leads to the excretion in the breath and from the skin of foul smelling selenium compounds. People taking inappropriately high selenium supplements are not pleasant companions.

Sodium and potassium. Sodium and potassium ions are important in generating electrical impulses in the nervous system, and both are dietary essentials. Except where salt losses in sweat are excessive, as may occur in the tropics, or during vigorous exercise, sodium deficiency is not a problem. Indeed, the main concern is that average intakes of sodium (mainly in table salt added to foods) are excessively high, and high intakes of sodium are associated with increased blood pressure and increased risk of stroke. While both sodium and potassium are found in most foods, fruits and vegetables are good sources of potassium with little sodium.

Vitamins

Eleven compounds are considered to be vitamins. Four (vitamins A, D, E, and K) are fat-soluble; the remainder are water-soluble and act mainly as coenzymes in various metabolic reactions. In addition, there are a small number of compounds that have clear metabolic functions in the body, but are not considered to be vitamins since they can be made in the body in adequate amounts. Such compounds include carnitine, choline, inositol, taurine, and ubiquinone (which is sometimes misleadingly sold as vitamin Q).

Vitamin A. Vitamin A has two very different functions in the body. It provides the visual pigment in the eye that is sensitive to light and leads to the initiation of a nerve impulse to the visual centres of the brain. It also acts like a hormone, binding to intracellular receptors, regulating the expression of genes, and controlling tissue differentiation during development. Vitamin A receptors with the vitamin bound are also essential for the actions of vitamin D and thyroid hormone.

There are two sources of vitamin A in the diet: preformed vitamin A in meat, and carotenes in red, yellow, and orange fruits and vegetables, as well as green leafy vegetables, which can be converted to vitamin A in the body. The name carotene comes from the fact that β-carotene was first isolated from carrots.

Vitamin A deficiency is the largest preventable cause of blindness world-wide. Deficiency is a major problem of public health, with 14 million children deficient and more than 190 million people at risk of deficiency.

Taken in excess, however, vitamin A is toxic. While there is a 12-fold difference between desirable levels of intake and the toxic threshold in adults, for children there is only a 3.5-fold difference. For pregnant women the difference is less than 5-fold; excess vitamin A causes fetal abnormalities, and pregnant women are advised not to eat liver and liver products, which are especially rich sources of the vitamin.

Vitamin D. Vitamin D is essential for the absorption of calcium from the diet, and hence for the maintenance of normal calcium metabolism and bone formation. As we have seen, deficiency leads to rickets in children and osteomalacia in adults. Rickets was a major problem of public health in many Northern countries until the introduction of vitamin D enrichment of infant foods in the 1940s. The vitamin is toxic in excess, and a small number of infants developed signs of vitamin D poisoning. As a result, the level of food enrichment was reduced, and up to 10 per cent of young children now show sub-clinical signs of deficiency.

Like vitamin A, vitamin D acts as a hormone, controlling gene expression. There is increasing evidence that in addition to its functions in calcium absorption and metabolism, it is important in regulating the expression of a large number of genes, and higher intakes of vitamin D than are considered to be adequate for bone health may provide protection against some cancers, type II diabetes, and possibly also obesity.

Apart from fortified foods, there are few dietary sources of vitamin D: oily fish (such as herring, salmon, and trout), eggs, and full-fat dairy produce (butter, cream, and cheese). The vitamin can also be synthesized in the skin when there is adequate sunlight exposure. In Northern countries, this is possible only in summertime, and there is considerable seasonal variation in the blood concentration of vitamin D. By the end of winter, the average blood concentration is only slightly higher than that seen in marginal deficiency.

While increased sunlight exposure provides a way of increasing vitamin D status without the problems of toxicity that might be seen if there was widespread excessive enrichment of foods, it also increases the risk of developing skin cancer. Because of the paucity of dietary sources, and the risks of excessive sunlight exposure, it is accepted that supplements are required for pregnant and lactating women, and people over the age of 65, to meet the recommended intake of 10 μg/day. There is evidence that higher intakes, 10–20 μg/day, have health benefits for all adults.

Vitamin E. Vitamin E functions as an antioxidant in cell membranes and plasma lipoproteins. Requirements vary depending on the intake of polyunsaturated fats, but dietary deficiency is extremely rare, since most oils that are rich sources of polyunsaturates are also rich sources of vitamin E. The antioxidant actions of vitamins E and C are related; oxidized vitamin E in cell membranes and plasma lipoproteins is reduced back to the active vitamin by reacting with vitamin C in the blood plasma and cytosol of the cell. Oxidized vitamin C can be reduced back to the active vitamin enzymically.

There is a considerable body of epidemiological evidence that high vitamin E status is associated with a lower risk of atherosclerosis and coronary heart disease. However, intervention trials have shown increased mortality among people taking high-dose supplements of vitamin E.

Vitamin K. Vitamin K is required for the synthesis of blood clotting proteins and proteins involved in the mineralization of bone. Dietary deficiency is rare, because vitamin K is present in plant oils and green leafy vegetables. Intestinal bacteria synthesize it, although it is not clear how much of this bacterial vitamin K is absorbed.

Deficiency of vitamin K leads to impaired blood clotting, and prolonged bleeding. The widely used anticoagulant drugs used to treat people at risk of blood clots, such as Warfarin, act as antagonists of vitamin K. The vitamin also acts to antagonize the actions of the anticoagulant drugs, and problems may arise when people taking anticoagulants either start to take vitamin K supplements, or stop taking them when their dose of anticoagulant has been increased to overcome the effect of high intakes of the vitamin.

Vitamin B₁. Vitamin B_1 (thiamin) acts as a coenzyme in a number of key reactions in carbohydrate and general energy-yielding metabolism, as well as having a role in nerve transmission. Deficiency of thiamin, leading to the disease of beriberi, was formerly common in the Far East after the introduction of steam-powered rice mills and the widespread use of polished rice—the vitamin is in the bran that is discarded when rice is milled. Potatoes, cereals, and meat are rich sources of thiamin; pork is an especially rich source.

Nowadays, deficiency occurs mainly in alcoholics with a poor food intake, because alcohol inhibits the absorption of the vitamin. In this case, deficiency causes brain damage, leading to the Wernicke-Korsakoff syndrome—loss of recent memory (although distant memory may be unimpaired) and neurological signs. Deficiency also occurs when people who have been starved for a period of time are given intravenous glucose without added thiamin. In this case (and sometimes in alcoholics) there are disturbances of carbohydrate metabolism leading to potentially life-threatening acidosis.

Vitamin B₂. Vitamin B_2 (riboflavin) acts as a coenzyme in a number of energy-yielding metabolic pathways. Deficiency is relatively common in some countries, but is rarely fatal. This is because as the intake of riboflavin falls, so the vitamin that is released when enzymes turn over is very efficiently salvaged and re-used.

Milk and dairy produce are important sources of riboflavin (as well as of calcium and protein), and riboflavin status reflects dairy consumption in many countries.

Niacin. Two compounds have the activity of the vitamin niacin: nicotinic acid and nicotinamide. They are interconvertible in the body, and the function of niacin is to provide the coenzyme nicotinamide adenine dinucleotide (NAD), which is involved in a very large number of oxidation and reduction reactions in the body. Meat, eggs, and fish provide significant amounts of preformed niacin, as does coffee; cereals are a poor source.

In addition to using the vitamin, NAD can be synthesized in the body from the essential amino acid tryptophan, and under normal conditions this probably meets requirements for niacin without the need for a dietary source of the preformed vitamin. Most foods, apart from maize and sorghum, contain significant amounts of tryptophan, and if protein needs are met, then so is the need for niacin.

Pellagra, the niacin deficiency disease, was a major public health problem in the southern USA until the middle of the 20th century, and in other areas of the world (especially Southern Africa) where maize provided the dietary staple, with little meat or other sources of tryptophan. The proteins of maize contain very little tryptophan, and, as in other cereals, most of the niacin in maize is chemically bound to carbohydrates and is not available for absorption. Pellagra was never a problem in Mexico, the original home of maize, because of the traditional method of preparing the grain. It was not ground into flour, but was soaked in (alkaline) lime water. This treatment liberates niacin from the otherwise unavailable complexes with carbohydrates.

Vitamin B_6. Vitamin B_6 is required for the action of a large number of enzymes involved in the metabolism of amino acids and in mobilization of the storage carbohydrate glycogen in liver and muscles. It has a separate function in regulating the activity of steroid hormones. Meat, fish, and legumes are good sources of vitamin B_6.

Deficiency of this vitamin leads to abnormalities of amino acid metabolism, and a number of studies suggest that although clinical deficiency disease is uncommon, marginal deficiency may occur in 10 per cent of the population in developed countries.

Studies in the 1960s suggested that high-dose oral contraceptive drugs led to vitamin B_6 deficiency. However, this was an artefact, and was in fact the result of oestrogen metabolites inhibiting an enzyme in tryptophan metabolism, leading to biochemical changes that falsely suggested B_6 deficiency. There are no such problems with modern low-dose oral contraceptives.

Some studies have suggested that relatively high doses of vitamin B_6 (50 to 100 mg/day) relieve the symptoms of premenstrual syndrome. There is little evidence of efficacy from controlled trials, but the vitamin is still prescribed and self-prescribed for premenstrual syndrome. There is some evidence that doses between 25 to 100 mg/day may lead to nerve damage; certainly this occurs with intakes above 200 g/day.

Folic acid (folate). Folic acid acts in a variety of reactions involving the transfer of one-carbon units from one compound onto another, including DNA synthesis and vitamin B_{12} metabolism. Deficiency is relatively common, leading to megaloblastic anaemia—the release into the bloodstream of immature red blood cell precursors. Legumes, fruits and vegetables, meat, and fish are all good sources of folate.

Supplements of folic acid of the order of 400 µg/day (in addition to the normal dietary intake) reduce the incidence of spina bifida and neural tube defect very considerably. The neural tube closes, and therefore the damage is done, before day 21 of pregnancy, which is before a woman knows she is pregnant. Therefore, in the UK and many other countries, women who are planning pregnancy are advised to start taking folic acid supplements before conception. The problem is, of course, that many pregnancies are unplanned.

A number of countries (including the USA and Canada) have therefore introduced mandatory fortification of flour with folic acid, and this has led to a significant decrease in the number of infants born with neural tube defects.

A relatively common genetic abnormality, affecting 10 per cent of the population, leads to a high blood concentration of the metabolic intermediate homocysteine, which is a factor in the development of atherosclerosis. The abnormal gene occurs in 17 per cent of people with atherosclerosis, but only 5 per cent of those without. High intakes of folic acid overcome the gene abnormality, and lead to reduction in the blood concentration of homocysteine. There is also some evidence that poor folic acid status is a factor in colorectal cancer.

There are a number of potential problems with widespread enrichment of foods with folic acid, which explain why many countries have not introduced mandatory enrichment of flour. As people age, their secretion of gastric acid decreases, and they are unable to release vitamin B_{12} from proteins in foods, leading to possible deficiency. Like folic acid deficiency, vitamin B_{12} deficiency causes megaloblastic anaemia, but it also causes irreversible nerve damage. A high intake of folic acid prevents the development of the anaemia, and elderly people with vitamin B_{12} deficiency will first present with the irreversible nerve damage rather than the reversible anaemia. High blood concentrations of folic acid also antagonize the actions of some of the anticonvulsant drugs used to treat epilepsy. Although poor folic acid status is associated with increased incidence of colorectal cancer, there is some evidence that high intakes of the vitamin by people who have benign precancerous polyps may accelerate the transition to cancer.

If the enrichment of flour with folic acid is to be made mandatory, there needs to be a careful balancing act between providing intakes that will have a significant effect on reducing the incidence of neural tube defects and intakes that will put the elderly at risk. The UK Food Standards Agency has advised that if mandatory enrichment were to be introduced, all voluntary enrichment of other foods would have to cease.

Vitamin B₁₂. Vitamin B_{12} is required for only two metabolic reactions, the most important of which is the folic acid dependent conversion of homocysteine to the amino acid methionine. As noted above, deficiency leads to megaloblastic anaemia, which is the result of trapping folic acid as a derivative that cannot be used without vitamin B_{12}, and irreversible nerve damage, which is the result of a deficiency of methionine in the nervous system. Because of this nerve damage, the condition is known as pernicious anaemia.

There are no plant sources of vitamin B_{12}, and strict vegetarians (Vegans) are at risk of dietary deficiency unless they take supplements made by bacterial fermentation (which are ethically acceptable to them). The richest sources are meat and fish, but eggs and milk provide significant amounts. From time to time there are suggestions that algae and fermented soya products contain vitamin B_{12}, but this is misleading. The legally required method of measuring vitamin B_{12} is by its ability to act as a growth factor for a specific strain of bacteria, but this also measures analogues of the vitamin that are growth factors for the bacteria, but do not have vitamin activity in human beings.

The absorption of vitamin B_{12} from foods requires the action of gastric acid to release the vitamin from proteins it is bound to. The vitamin then binds to a small protein (intrinsic factor) that is secreted in the stomach, and the intrinsic factor–vitamin complex is then absorbed in the small intestine. Failure of gastric acid and intrinsic factor secretion (achlorhydria), or the production of auto-immune antibodies against either intrinsic factor or the cells in the stomach that secrete it, leads to failure to absorb the vitamin, and the development of pernicious anaemia. It is treated by injection of the vitamin, or, in cases where the problem is failure to secrete intrinsic factor, oral doses of intrinsic factor. The reduction in gastric acid secretion without loss of intrinsic factor secretion that is seen with increasing age impairs the absorption of dietary vitamin B_{12} bound to proteins, but not the absorption of crystalline vitamin B_{12} from supplements.

Biotin. Biotin acts in a small number of metabolic reactions, and also has a role in controlling cell division and proliferation. The vitamin is widespread in foods, and deficiency has only been reported in a small number of people who consumed abnormally large amounts of uncooked egg white (typically a dozen or more raw eggs a day for several years). The protein avidin in egg white binds biotin so that it is not available for absorption. However, when the egg is cooked, avidin is denatured and can no longer bind biotin.

Pantothenic acid. Pantothenic acid (sometimes called vitamin B_5) acts as the coenzyme for synthesis and metabolism of fatty acids, and a number of other reactions. The vitamin is widely distributed in foods and deficiency is unknown except in specific depletion studies.

Experimental studies of animals that are deprived of pantothenic acid have found that they lose their fur pigmentation, and so the vitamin was at one time known as the 'anti-grey hair factor'. There is no evidence that supplements of pantothenic acid prevent the normal greying of hair with ageing, and there is certainly no evidence that adding it to shampoo has any beneficial effect.

Prisoners of war in the Far East in the Second World War developed a painful condition known as the burning foot syndrome, which was tentatively attributed to pantothenic acid deficiency. However, for obvious reasons, they were not subject to experiments in order to determine if pantothenic acid was the problem. Levels were replenished with yeast extract, this being a rich source of all B vitamins.

Vitamin C. Vitamin C acts as a water-soluble antioxidant, both in its own right and by reducing oxidized vitamin E back to the

84

active vitamin. It also acts in a small number of enzymes, including those involved in the synthesis of the connective tissue proteins collagen and elastin and the neurotransmitters and hormones noradrenaline and adrenaline. The main sources are fruits and vegetables.

Deficiency leads to the disease scurvy, which is characterized by poor healing of wounds, loosening of the teeth and inflammation of the gums, small haemorrhages under the skin, and intense bone pain. All of these can be attributed to impaired synthesis of connective tissue proteins. In addition there are psychological changes ('scurvy' means 'ill-tempered'), which can be attributed to impaired synthesis of noradrenaline and adrenaline.

Vitamin C is generally considered to have very low toxicity, and relatively large doses (up to several grams per day) can be tolerated, although very large doses may cause gastro-intestinal upset due to bacterial fermentation of unabsorbed vitamin. At intakes over about 100 mg/day, the vitamin is excreted in the urine. It is an acid, and acidifies the urine. This may have the beneficial effect of increasing the solubility of phosphates in the urine, and so reducing the formation of phosphate kidney stones. However, cysteine, oxalic acid, uric acid, and xanthine are less soluble in acidic urine, and high doses of vitamin C will increase the formation of kidney stones containing these compounds.

Phytochemicals and nutraceuticals

A wide variety of compounds in fruits and vegetables may have beneficial effects in the body, although they are not considered to be dietary essentials, and therefore are not classified as vitamins. Collectively they are known as phytochemicals or nutraceuticals.

The carotenes (the pigments of yellow, orange, and red fruits and vegetables), the anthocyanins (the pigments of red, purple, and blue fruits and vegetables) and the polyphenols or bioflavonoids, found in a wide variety of fruits and vegetables, and also in tea and red wine, are all potential antioxidants, and may have other beneficial effects.

Glucosinolates, glycosides, and sulphur-containing compounds from a variety of foods, especially brassicas (cabbages, cauliflower, sprouts, broccoli, etc.) modify the synthesis and activity of enzymes that metabolize a variety of foreign compounds. Many of these foreign compounds in foods are potential carcinogens, and increasing the activity of the enzymes that metabolize them may reduce the risk of cancer. These compounds are also capable of modifying the metabolism of prescription medication, and reducing its efficacy. The only potentially serious such interaction is with compounds found in grapefruit, and many prescription medicines carry a warning not to consume grapefruit or grapefruit juice while taking the medicine.

Terpenes in citrus oil, ginger, and other spices inhibit the synthesis of cholesterol, and may be useful in the treatment of elevated blood cholesterol. Squalene is an intermediate in cholesterol synthesis. It occurs in relatively large amounts in olive oil, and again acts to inhibit the synthesis of cholesterol. While this may be beneficial, it is also possible that it will be metabolized onwards to cholesterol, so negating some of the potential benefit.

A number of compounds in soya beans have anti-oestrogenic activity, and may be beneficial in prevention of hormone-dependent cancer of the breast, uterus, and prostate. They act by binding to the oestrogen receptor in competition with oestrogens, but they only activate the receptor weakly. Some studies show that habitual consumption of soya products reduces the risk of breast cancer, but others have shown no significant effect.

How much is enough—and can we have too much?

Estimating requirements for vitamins and establishing desirable levels of intake depends on experiments in which volunteers are maintained on a diet that is otherwise adequate, but lacking the vitamin under study, until there is a detectable metabolic abnormality that is a sign of early vitamin deficiency. Levels are then replenished by gradually increasing doses of the deficient vitamin until the metabolic abnormality is just normalized.

Figure 4 shows the results of such an experiment. There is a range of individual requirements around the average, and in most cases there is a statistically normal distribution. This means that a range of ± 2 x standard deviation around the average will include 95 per cent of the population. An intake of average requirement +2 x standard deviations will therefore be greater than the requirement of 97.5 per cent of the population. This is selected as a reference intake to be used in food labelling, in planning meals for institutions, and in assessing the adequacy or otherwise of populations. The reference intake is greater than the requirements of 97.5 per cent of the population, so if an individual has an intake below the reference intake, this does not mean that he or she is deficient.

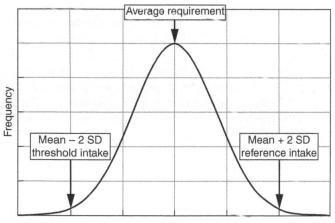

4. **The derivation of reference intakes for nutrients**

This reference intake is known by a variety of names in different countries:

RDA—recommended daily (or dietary) amount (or allowance);
RNI—reference nutrient intake;
PRI—population reference intake;
DV—daily value (used in USA for food labelling, based on a
    notional 2,000 kcal diet).

The term 'reference nutrient intake' (RNI) was coined in the 1991 report on nutrient requirements of the UK Department of Health, by parallel with clinical chemistry, where this 95 per cent range around the average value of a metabolite is known as the 'reference range' for a given group of the population. It was considered inappropriate to call this a 'recommendation', since the intake figures do not apply to an individual, or to call it 'an allowance'. A further reason for this choice of terminology is that this is the amount per day on average, and not a precise daily amount. The 1993 report of the EU Scientific Committee on Food coined the term 'population reference intake' to emphasize that the figures refer to populations, not to individuals. However, the term 'recommended daily (or dietary) amount (or allowance)' (RDA) is still used in food labelling in the EU.

Tables of reference intakes published by different national and international authorities include separate values for men and women, for different ages and for pregnancy and lactation. The values in different tables vary. Sometimes this is because a later expert group has access to more recent experimental data, and sometimes because different expert groups interpret the same experimental evidence differently. Table 7 shows the values that are used in food labelling in the USA and the EU.

It was noted above that some vitamins and minerals are toxic if taken in excess. Table 7 also shows the 'tolerable upper levels' of habitual consumption that have been set by the US Institute of

Medicine and the European Food Safety Authority, on the basis of the highest level of intake that is not known to cause any adverse effects, modified by a safety factor where appropriate.

Table 7. Labelling reference intakes and tolerable upper levels of habitual intake of vitamins and minerals for adults

Vitamin	Reference intake		Tolerable upper level	
	US Daily Value	EU RDA	US Institute of Medicine	European Food Safety Authority
A	900 µg	800 µg	3000 µg	3000 µg
D	10 µg	5 µg	100 µg	100 µg
E	15 mg	10 mg	1000 µg	300 mg
K	80 µg	–	–	–
B_1	1.5 mg	1.4 mg	–	–
B_2	1.7 mg	1.6 mg	–	–
Niacin	20 mg	18 mg	35 mg	10 mg nicotinic acid 900 mg nicotinamide
B_6	2 mg	2 mg	100 mg	25 mg
Folate	400 µg	200 µg	1000 µg	1000 µg
B_{12}	6 µg	1 µg	–	–
Biotin	300 µg	150 µg	–	–
Pantothenic acid	10 mg	6 mg	–	–
C	60 mg	60 mg	2000 mg	–
Mineral				
Calcium	1000 mg	700 mg	2500 mg	2500 mg

(*continued*)

Vitamins and minerals

Table 7. Continued

Minerals	Reference intake		Tolerable upper level	
	US Daily Value	EU RDA	US Institute of Medicine	European Food Safety Authority
Copper	2 mg	1.1 mg	10 mg	5 mg
Fluoride	–	–	10 mg	7 mg
Iodine	150 µg	130 µg	1100 µg	600 µg
Iron	18 mg	9 mg	45 mg	–
Magnesium	400 mg	–	350 mg	250 mg
Manganese	2 mg	–	11 mg	–
Molybdenum	75 µg	–	2000 µg	500 µg
Phosphorus	1000 mg	550 mg	3000 mg	–
Selenium	70 µg	55 µg	400 µg	300 µg
Vanadium	–	–	1.8 mg	–
Zinc	15 mg	9.5 mg	40 mg	25 mg
Sodium	2400 mg	–	–	–

From data reported by: EFSA Panel on Dietetic Products, Nutrition and Allergies (NDA) (2012). 'Scientific Opinion on the Tolerable Upper Intake Level of vitamin D'. *EFSA Journal* 10(7): 2813 (available at: <http://www.efsa.europa.eu/en/publications.htm>). Scientific Committee for Food (1993). *Nutrient and Energy Intakes for the European Community*; Commission of the European Communities, Luxembourg, EFSA (European Food Safety Authority) (2006). Scientific Committee on Food Scientific Panel on Dietetic Products, Nutrition and Allergies (2006). *Tolerable Upper Intake Levels for Vitamins and Minerals*. European Food Safety Authority (available from <http://www.efsa.europa.eu/en/publications. htm>). Standing Committee on the Scientific Evaluation of Dietary Reference Intakes, Food and Nutrition Board, Institute of Medicine (1997). 'Dietary Reference Intakes for Calcium, Phosphorus, Magnesium, Vitamin D and Fluoride'; (1998).'Dietary Reference Intakes for Thiamin, Riboflavin, Niacin, Vitamin B_6, Folate, Vitamin B_{12}, Pantothenic Acid, Biotin and Choline'; (2000). 'Dietary Reference Intakes for Vitamin C, Vitamin E, Selenium and Carotenoids; (2001). 'Dietary Reference Intakes for Vitamin A, Vitamin K, Arsenic, Boron, Chromium, Copper, Iodine, Iron, Manganese, Molybdenum, Nickel, Silicon, Vanadium and Zinc'. National Academy Press, Washington, DC. <www.fda.gov/food/guidanceregulation/ gluidancedocumentsregulatoryinformation/lebellingnutriton/ucm664928.htm>

Chapter 8
Functional foods, superfoods, and supplements

Functional foods

Functional foods are defined as foods that contain one or more added ingredients to provide a positive health benefit, over and above the normal functions of food to provide nutrients and satisfy hunger. This definition excludes vitamins and minerals added to foods to replace losses in manufacture.

The concept of functional foods was developed in Japan in the 1980s, with a formal definition of 'foods for specified health use' (FOSHU), accompanied by a regulatory system to approve the statements made on labels and in advertising, based on scientific evaluation of the evidence of efficacy and safety. While there may be good evidence of *potential* benefits of some functional foods, and well conducted trials show improvement in indices of physiological function (biomarkers) and risk factors, as yet there is little evidence of improved health or increased lifespan in most cases.

When a vitamin or mineral deficiency is widespread in a population, a common approach is to enrich or fortify a staple food. The problem here is that if enrichment is voluntary, so that consumers have a choice of whether to buy the fortified or unfortified product, it is likely that the most vulnerable groups of the population will not be reached. However, if enrichment is mandatory then political problems of freedom of choice arise. It is noteworthy that despite the excellent evidence that fluoride reduces dental decay very significantly, fluoridation of water supplies is not universal in Britain, because of (unfounded) fears of 'mass medication'.

Two examples of functional foods for which there is some evidence of efficacy are foods that modify the intestinal bacterial population, and foods that reduce the absorption of cholesterol.

Intestinal bacteria—prebiotics, probiotics, and synbiotics. It is a sobering thought that we host ten times more bacteria in the intestinal tract than there are cells in the human body. Some of the 100 or more species are pathogenic, some are harmless, and some (especially the lactic acid producing bacteria) are beneficial, producing a variety of compounds that prevent the growth of pathogenic organisms. They ferment dietary fibre to provide short-chain fatty acids that are the preferred fuel for intestinal mucosal cells and may have anti-cancer activity.

The main lactic acid producing bacteria of interest are *Lactobacillus* and *Bifidobacterium* spp., and there is some evidence of beneficial effects of lactic acid bacteria in controlling allergies, preventing or curing constipation, and generally maintaining gastro-intestinal health. These are the bacteria that are present in probiotic yoghurts. An alternative approach to modifying intestinal bacteria is the consumption of undigested carbohydrates (dietary fibre and starch that is resistant to digestion) that provide a substrate for fermentation by the probiotic bacteria, and are therefore known as prebiotics. The combination of the two, probiotic bacteria and prebiotic carbohydrates, is known as a synbiotic.

There is good evidence for the effects of some prebiotics in alleviating constipation. The evidence is less good for the prevention of colon cancer, intestinal infection, and recurrence of inflammatory bowel disease, but a number of trials have suggested that prebiotics can prevent colonization of the intestinal tract with pathogens.

Plant sterols and stanols to lower serum cholesterol. Average daily intakes of cholesterol from the diet are between 300 to 600 mg/day; in addition to this, some 2,000 mg of cholesterol is secreted each day in the bile, much of which is reabsorbed. This means that anything that will reduce cholesterol absorption from the small intestine will have a much larger effect on whole body cholesterol (and hence serum cholesterol) than would be expected from the dietary intake alone.

Analogues of cholesterol, such as the plant sterol β-sitosterol and the stanols, inhibit the enzymes that convert cholesterol to cholesterol esters in the intestinal mucosa, for absorption, so that less enters the circulation. Unesterified cholesterol is actively exported from the mucosal cells back into the gut. There is abundant evidence that consumption of plant sterols and stanols lowers blood cholesterol, and the effect is additive to that of statins, the drugs that inhibit cholesterol synthesis. Plant sterols and stanols are found in moderate amounts in fruits, vegetables, nuts, and vegetable oils. A variety of low fat spreads, yoghurts, drinks, and cream cheeses enriched with plant sterols and stanols have been marketed.

Superfoods

The concept of 'superfoods' was developed in the USA in 2003–4 and was introduced in Britain by an article in the *Daily Mail* in December 2005. Superfoods are ordinary foods that are especially rich in nutrients or antioxidants and other potentially protective compounds, including polyunsaturated fatty acids and dietary fibre.

A web search for 'superfoods' gives the following list:

> almonds, apples, avocado, baked beans, bananas, beetroot, blueberries,
> Brazil nuts, broccoli, Brussels sprouts, cabbage, carrots, cocoa,
> cranberries, flax seeds, garlic, ginger, kiwi, mango, olive oil, onions,
> oranges, peppers, pineapple, pumpkin, red grapes, salmon, soy,
> spinach, strawberries, sunflower seeds, sweet potato, tea, tomatoes,
> watercress, whole grain seeded bread, whole grains, wine, yoghurt.

There are very few surprises in this list. Most of these are foods
that we know are nutrient dense—with a high content of vitamins
and minerals/1,000 kcal. The nuts, seeds, and olive oil are an
exception, but they are all good sources of polyunsaturated fatty
acids and vitamins E and K.

The labelling and marketing of the foods as superfoods seems
disingenuous (or a clever marketing strategy), but if such marketing
leads people to eat more fruit and vegetables and to reduce their
saturated fat, salt, and sugar intake then it can only help to reinforce
the message about the prudent diet discussed in Chapter 5.

Supplements

The term 'nutritional supplements' covers a very wide range of
preparations whose common denominator is that they are
regarded as foods rather than medicines, and in most countries
are regulated under food legislation rather than laws relating to
medicines. In the USA specified health claims are permitted by
the Food and Drug Administration (FDA), but manufacturers are
also permitted to make further claims, provided that these bear a
note to the effect that the claims have not been evaluated by FDA,
and that the product is not intended to diagnose, treat, cure, or
prevent any disease. In Europe, the European Food Safety
Authority (EFSA) has begun the lengthy process of evaluating the
evidence for health claims submitted by manufacturers of foods
and supplements, in order to draw up a list of permitted claims.

Arguably, the least controversial supplements are multi-vitamin and mineral mixtures that provide about 100 per cent of the reference intake per day. This is already an unnecessary amount for most people, since they will have at least some intake from their foods. A number of surveys in developed countries show that average intakes of vitamins and minerals from foods are adequate to meet requirements. Of course, for people with a low food intake (and this will include many elderly people with low energy expenditure, and therefore low food intake) such supplements may well be advisable, or at least a prudent precaution. Similarly, for people whose diet is relatively poor, supplements are advisable. Unfortunately, most surveys show that supplements are purchased mainly by people whose diet is already adequate, not by those for whom they might be desirable.

Supplements that provide higher amounts of vitamins and minerals are a cause for concern. As discussed in Chapter 7, excessive intakes can be harmful. It is highly unlikely that a manufacturer would deliberately market a supplement containing a dangerously high amount of a nutrient. However, it would be possible to achieve an undesirably high, and even hazardous, intake by taking a number of different supplements, each of which provided a high, but safe, amount of a vitamin or mineral. This is especially a concern for vitamin A, where the margin between adequacy and potential toxicity is relatively small—especially for young children and pregnant women (see Table 7).

There is a good basis of evidence to recommend some single nutrient supplements. As discussed in Chapter 7, folic acid supplements of 400 µg/day are recommended for women planning pregnancy and vitamin D supplements of 10 to 20 µg per day are advisable for pregnant women and the elderly, since it is unlikely that they will meet the reference intake from the few foods that are rich sources of the vitamin. Indeed, there is increasing evidence for a benefit of vitamin D supplements for everyone living in temperate regions with little sunlight exposure.

Long-chain polyunsaturated fatty acids, as found in fish oils, provide protection against cardiovascular disease. For people who do not like oily fish, or eat it only rarely, supplements of fish oil will be beneficial. People whose diet is poor in fruit and vegetables will probably benefit from vitamin C supplements, and there is some (relatively weak) evidence that supplements of vitamin C may alleviate the symptoms of the common cold.

There is considerably less evidence, if any at all, for the benefits of other single nutrient supplements. As discussed in Chapter 5, relatively high-dose antioxidant supplements, especially carotene and vitamin E, are associated with a higher risk of death. It is certainly difficult to justify supplements of individual amino acids. Nevertheless, many single nutrient supplements, or preparations containing a small group of related nutrients, are widely available to be bought—both over the counter and by mail order/online.

One suggestion for regulating the market in nutritional supplements, which has not met with approval from any of the regulatory agencies, is to consider them in three groups.

Supplements containing nutritionally relevant amounts of nutrients (perhaps up to five to ten times the recommended daily amount (RDA) could be readily available over the counter, as at present, and be considered to be foods.

Supplements containing about ten to 50 times the RDA, where there is some risk of excessive intake, especially if you are taking more than one product, should be considered to be medicinal compounds rather than foods, and should be sold by qualified pharmacists, who can ask about other supplements and medicines you are taking.

Supplements containing more than about 50 times the RDA, where there might be a real risk of adverse effects of a high intake should be available only on prescription, since part of medical education includes learning how to balance the risks and benefits of treatment. There may well be some people who would benefit from a high dose of a given nutrient, even though there is a potential hazard to their health from the supplement.

As discussed in Chapter 3, there is little evidence for the efficacy of protein supplements marketed to athletes and sportspeople, and there may be undeclared ingredients such as steroids in some supplements that are banned in competitive sports. Creatine is often marketed as an ergogenic aid to improve sports performance. The rationale is that creatine (as its phosphate) provides a reserve to replenish ATP in muscle. Creatine is made in the body from amino acids and there is little evidence that supplements are effective in increasing performance, although a few studies do suggest benefits for such sports as arm wrestling, which require very short bursts of very high intensity muscle activity. Similarly, although carnitine is essential for uptake of fatty acids and their use as metabolic fuel in muscle, it can be synthesized in the body, and there is no evidence that supplements improve muscle function or athletic performance. There is little evidence that supplements of fish oils, containing ω-3 polyunsaturated fatty acids, have any beneficial effect on mental concentration or intelligence once requirements have been met from foods.

Many herbal preparations are marketed and regulated as nutritional supplements, although some are permitted as medical products with claims based on traditional use for treating various conditions. Some will indeed be effective—after all, many of the conventional medicines in use today have been derived from traditional herbal medicine, and many herbal preparations contain pharmacologically active compounds. Some, of course, may also be toxic, or may be contaminated with toxic metals because of where they were grown.

There is a need for caution in purchasing any nutritional supplement. If you buy products from a reputable manufacturer you can be reasonably sure that they have good quality control and laboratory facilities; that they analyse each batch of ingredients bought from suppliers; and can trace each batch of ingredients into each batch of their final products. By contrast, if you go online to buy supplements, while you may be lucky, the chances are that you will buy from a company that does not have its own laboratory facilities, and does not keep precise records of each batch of ingredients and products. They may be buying from their suppliers in good faith, but they cannot be sure that what they are selling meets appropriate standards of purity and safety.

If you follow the guidelines for a healthy diet discussed in Chapter 5, a varied, moderate diet will meet nutrient requirements for most people. It is important to avoid extreme or radical diets, and to be wary of bold claims that are sometimes made about foods. If you are healthy, then eat when you are hungry but stop before becoming unpleasantly full; and drink when you are thirsty, but there is no need for an excessive fluid intake.

Glossary

amino acid A compound with both an amino ($-NH_2$) and a carboxylic acid ($-COOH$) group attached to the α-carbon. Proteins are composed of amino acids.

atherosclerosis The accumulation of fatty deposits in blood vessels, leading to reduction of the size of the blood vessels. Atherosclerosis in the coronary arteries is the commonest cause of ischaemic heart attacks.

basal metabolic rate (BMR) The energy expenditure by the body at complete rest, but not asleep, in the post-prandial (i.e. after eating) state.

body mass index (BMI) The ratio of body weight/height^2 (kg/m^2). A person with a BMI over 25 is considered to be overweight, and over 30 to be obese.

carbohydrate Compounds of carbon, hydrogen, and oxygen in the ratio $C_nH_{2n}O_n$ The dietary carbohydrates are sugars, starches, and non-starch polysaccharides.

catabolism Metabolic reactions resulting in the breakdown of complex molecules to simpler products, commonly oxidation to carbon dioxide and water, linked to the phosphorylation of ADP to ATP.

enzyme A protein that acts as a catalyst in a metabolic reaction.

international units (iu) Before vitamins and other substances were purified, their potency was expressed in arbitrary, but standardized, units of biological activity. Now this measurement is obsolete, but vitamins A, D, and E are still sometimes quoted in iu.

lipid A general term including fats and oils (triacylglycerols), phospholipids, and steroids.

lower reference nutrient intake (LRNI) An intake of a nutrient below which it is unlikely that physiological needs will be met or metabolic integrity be maintained.

metabolic fuel Those dietary components which are oxidized as a source of metabolic energy fats, carbohydrates, proteins, and alcohol.

metabolism The processes of interconversion of chemical compounds in the body.

organic Chemically, all compounds of carbon, other than simple carbonate and bicarbonate salts, are called 'organic', since they were originally discovered in living matter. Also used to describe foods grown under specified conditions without the use of fertilizers, pesticides, etc.

physical activity ratio (PAR) Energy expenditure in a given activity, expressed as a ratio of the basal metabolic rate.

physical activity level (PAL) Energy expenditure, averaged over 24 hours, expressed as a ratio of the basal metabolic rate. The sum of the physical activity ratio x time spent for each activity during the day.

RDA Recommended daily (or dietary) allowance (or amount) of a nutrient. An intake of the nutrient two standard deviations above the observed mean requirement, and hence greater than the requirements of 97.5 per cent of the population.

RNI Reference nutrient intake, a term introduced in the 1992 UK Tables of Dietary Reference Values. An intake of the nutrient two standard deviations above the observed mean requirement, and hence greater than the requirements of 97.5 per cent of the population.

saturated An organic compound in which all carbon atoms are joined by single bonds, as opposed to unsaturated compounds with carbon—carbon double bonds. A saturated compound contains the maximum possible proportion of hydrogen.

standard deviation A statistical measure of the scatter of results around the average or mean value.

unsaturated An organic compound containing one or more carbon—carbon double bonds, and therefore less than the possible maximum proportion of hydrogen.

Nutrition

Further reading

Bender, D. A. (2014) *Introduction to Nutrition and Metabolism*, 5th edition, CRC Press, Boca Raton, Florida.
Gibney, M. J., Lanham-New, S. A., Cassidy A., and Vorster, H. H. (2009) *Introduction to Human Nutrition*, 2nd edition, The Nutrition Society Textbook series, Wiley-Blackwell, Chichester.

Some useful websites

British Nutrition Foundation <http://www.nutrition.org.uk/>
European Food Safety Authority <http://www.efsa.europa.eu/>
Food Safety Authority of Ireland <http://www.fsai.ie/>
Food Standards Agency <http://www.food.gov.uk/>
Scientific Advisory Committee on Nutrition <http://www.sacn.gov.uk/>
US Food and Drug Administration <http://www.fda.gov/>

Index

Nutrition

W

Index

Expand your collection of
VERY SHORT INTRODUCTIONS

ONLINE CATALOGUE
A Very Short Introduction

Our online catalogue is designed to make it easy to find your ideal Very Short Introduction. View the entire collection by subject area, watch author videos, read sample chapters, and download reading guides.

SOCIAL MEDIA
Very Short Introduction

Join our community
www.oup.com/vsi

- Join us online at the official Very Short Introductions
  Facebook page.
- Access the thoughts and musings of our authors with our
  online **blog**.
- Sign up for our monthly **e-newsletter** to receive information
  on all new titles publishing that month.
- Browse the full range of Very Short Introductions online.
- Read **extracts** from the Introductions for free.
- Visit our library of **Reading Guides**. These guides, written by our
  expert authors will help you to question again, why you think
  what you think.
- If you are a teacher or lecturer you can order inspection
  copies quickly and simply via our website.